PRAISE FOR *THE GARDEN WITHIN*

"The book you are holding in your hands contains wisdom, insight, and revelation that will revolutionize your life. Dr. Anita is not only a brilliant trauma therapist but she also has a pastoral heart that desires for every person to thrive and flourish in life. *The Garden Within* offers a biblical model of well-being. It clarifies how we were created to function spiritually, emotionally, mentally, and biologically. It debunks long-held beliefs and misconceptions that limit and contain our growth, and it unveils the strength, beauty, and importance of our emotions. The psalmist wrote in Proverbs 4:23 that the heart is the source of life, and this book proves that to be true. This is the faith and mental health book you've been waiting for."

—Christine Caine, founder of A21 and Propel Women

"*The Garden Within* by Dr. Anita Phillips is a blueprint that will empower you to defy the odds. Dr. Anita's dynamic bilingual capacity—translating seamlessly between the languages of Scripture and psychology in ways that haven't been heard before—is a gift. This is a paradigm-shifting book. You will truly be blessed and enriched by this God-inspired, practical, and personalized ministry tool."

—Bishop T. D. Jakes, CEO of TDJ Enterprises
and *New York Times* bestselling author

"I love Dr. Anita Phillips and the gift that God has given her to bring transformation. Too often, when trying to bridge the gap between the Bible and modern psychology, we're offered only secular ideas. This book is different. In *The Garden Within* Dr. Anita provides the revelation and education we need to live the abundant life God has for all of us. Prepare to be transformed both emotionally and spiritually."

—CeCe Winans, Grammy Award–winning
gospel artist and author of *Believe for It*

"Emotion is a gift from God, but it's a gift the enemy wants to steal, kill, and destroy. The good news? You can end the war with your emotions, and Dr. Anita Phillips shows you how! This book is like the healing balm of Gilead. It will heal you from the inside out."

—Mark Batterson, *New York Times* bestselling author of *The Circle Maker*

"Beautifully written and filled with wisdom, Dr. Anita takes us on a journey to deeply connect with ourselves and God while discovering the daily power of faith, hope, and love. *The Garden Within* is an instant favorite."

—Victoria Osteen, copastor of Lakewood Church and author

"This is a book for such a time as this. Dr. Anita's insights into what Scripture says about emotions provide a rich and refined perspective on this often-misunderstood topic. We need tools like this to combat the trauma that the world's chaos has invoked. This is a must-read for anyone seeking a deeper understanding of the intersection of faith and mental health."

—Latasha Morrison, author of
New York Times bestseller *Be the Bridge*

"Dr. Anita Phillips has been a trailblazer in guiding us toward embracing our emotional health with exceptional expertise. In an era when the significance of emotional well-being takes center stage in discussions, I wholeheartedly rely on her to navigate us toward practical and achievable solutions for healing and vitality. *The Garden Within* is an indispensable resource that we all need, and I greatly appreciate Dr. Anita's fearlessness in sharing her own life experiences throughout its pages."

—Dr. Dharius Daniels, author of *Your Purpose Is Calling*

"Dr. Anita Phillips has penned one of the most necessary books of our time. *The Garden Within* is a personal, powerful, and practical guide for all who understand the connection of their faith and mental health. Her unique ability to bring clarity to the intersectionality of theology, psychology, biology, and botany is only the beginning of helping us all move toward the necessary journey of wholeness. This book will change your life and I highly recommend it to you and everyone you love."

—Bishop Joseph Warren Walker III,
pastor of Mount Zion Church Nashville and International
Presiding Bishop of Full Gospel Baptist Church Fellowship

"*The Garden Within* by Dr. Anita Phillips has put me back on the couch in the most healing, reflective way! As a mental health advocate, and someone who has battled severe depression, my hope has been strengthened. I truly believe any person reading this book will also be strengthened, enlightened, and possibly convicted. Dr. Anita Phillips is one of the few that merges mental health and the word of God, eliminating stigma and igniting compassion for yourself or a person you may know who has a mental illness. If you're like me, you will be ready to lay prostrate during the book's introduction!"

—Michelle Williams, singer, author, and mental health advocate

"Revolutionary. Healing. A road map to living as we've been created to live. In the pages of this book, my dear friend Dr. Anita Phillips beautifully opens up our eyes to the truth about our emotional well-being and spiritual power. This book will be a timeless classic and go-to guide for people ready to heal, move forward, and flourish."

—Hosanna Wong, international speaker, spoken word artist, and author of *You Are More Than You've Been Told*

"In her book, *The Garden Within*, Dr. Anita Phillips skillfully explains the depths of our emotions and the power they hold in our lives as followers of Christ. With her expertise as a trauma therapist and her understanding of the human experience, Dr. Phillips masterfully guides the reader toward cultivating a powerfully 'free' life that aligns with the divine intentions of our Creator. What sets this book apart is Dr. Phillips's unwavering focus on Christ as the ultimate Gardener of our souls. She reminds us that it is through our emotional experiences, both pleasant and painful, that we can ultimately harness our spiritual power. This book will cause you to view and accept your emotions in a whole new way!"

—John K. Jenkins Sr., senior pastor at First Baptist Church of Glenarden

"Dr. Anita is someone who has made a huge impact on our lives. Her insight into the intersection between the Bible and mental health science is second to none. Reading this book was a balm to our hearts. Everyone who has hurt, pain, or trauma in their past should read this book!"

—Johnny and Jeni Baker, global executive directors of Celebrate Recovery

"Dr. Anita Phillips is a rare and desperately needed voice of sound biblical practice and trauma-informed care. She is a gifted writer, orator, clinician, and teacher. The concepts from *The Garden Within* will root your spirit in healthier soil. This book and her practice are for people who want to find greater and more complete healing. In a world filled with gimmicks and self-help guides, this is *not* that. *The Garden Within* provides specific instructional tools for hope, growth, and blooming."

—Nelba Márquez-Greene, LMFT, Sandy Hook parent, and founder of the Ana Grace Project

"For too many years we have been made to believe that our emotions are a weakness that must be denied. But in *The Garden Within*, Dr. Anita Phillips lovingly reminds us that the only way to experience true strength is to recognize our feelings for what they are: tools given by God with which to excavate the soil of our heart. This book is a healing balm for a generation."
—Nona Jones, tech executive, preacher, and author of *Killing Comparison*

"Becoming aware of the garden within is like discovering a source of much needed oxygen for your soul that you didn't even know existed. Dr Anita brilliantly reveals the 'prescription' to connect the parts of us that God never designed to function separately. The book becomes a bridge between our emotional, mental, and spiritual health that clearly articulates the road map to healing and wholeness. I've known Dr. Anita for several years and have been personally challenged and transformed by this message. The book you hold has the potential to revolutionize your life—you won't be able to put it down!"
—Dr. Donna Pisani, cofounder of Capital City Church and the Circle of 12 and author of *The Power of Not Yet*

"As someone who has tried to 'stuff' and ignore emotions throughout my life, I found this message that bridges mental health and faith completely freeing and transformative. Dr. Anita's new book, *The Garden Within*, leads and guides you on a liberating journey where you don't have to ignore your emotions to experience a revolution in your life—you just need to overthrow the lies you have believed about them."
—Nick Nilson, author and associate pastor at Lakewood Church

"Emotional health seems to be a key phrase these days. We all want it, but so many don't know how to get there. In *The Garden Within*, my friend Dr. Anita Phillips has written a groundbreaking book that connects our emotional well-being to our minds and our bodies. As a trauma therapist—who herself experienced trauma—she communicates with compassion and truth as she guides us on this journey. This book needs to be on everyone's shelf. The wisdom contained within is truly remarkable."
—Holly Wagner, cofounder of Oasis Church, founder of She Rises, and author of *Find Your Brave*

THE GARDEN WITHIN

WHERE THE WAR WITH YOUR EMOTIONS ENDS
& YOUR MOST POWERFUL LIFE BEGINS

DR. ANITA PHILLIPS

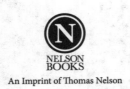

NELSON
BOOKS

An Imprint of Thomas Nelson

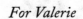

For Valerie

CONTENTS

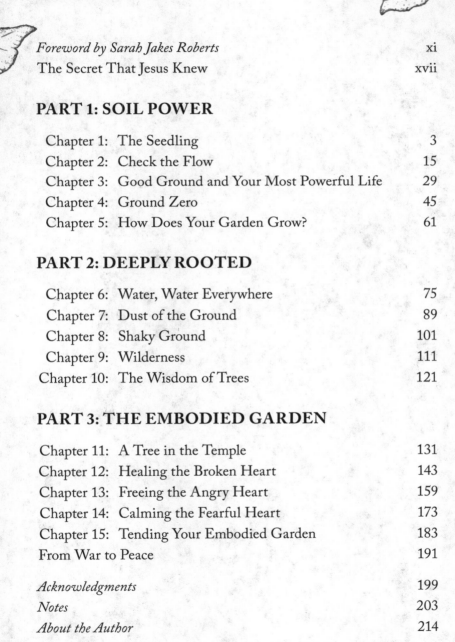

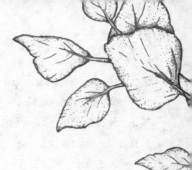

FOREWORD

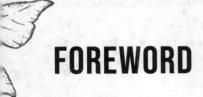

by Sarah Jakes Roberts

Dr. Anita Phillips and I occupied the same space at countless dinner parties and navigated several backstage halls, but we never shared more than a polite smile and quick salutation. I can't even pinpoint when we went from two ships passing in a green room to colleagues, friends, and, finally, sisters. All I know for sure is that I intentionally keep my circle small, but by divine providence it expanded before I knew it, and, frankly, without my permission. God knew the only way to get past my guards was to catch me by surprise. It might help for you to get to know me a bit before diving into how I became so guarded in the first place.

I never felt that I had faith like Sarah, courage like Ruth, wisdom like Esther, or obedience like Mary. These heroines of biblical virtue felt so far from who I was that oceans could have separated us. I grew up in church but never admitted that I felt out of touch. Of course, anyone observing my life's trajectory could see it clear as day. I felt safer in the back corner of a room than standing in front where all could see me. My desire to stay off the grid was not a result of my teenage pregnancy at thirteen. I was isolating long before then because I was battling so much internally.

I was confused, lost, angry, and lonely. I wanted to feel better, and I wasn't convinced that the solution could be found in the pews. Only after a few heartbreaks, a run-in with the police, and a divorce did I learn that the streets weren't offering much peace either. Surrendering was my only option, and that's what I did. I decided to make my relationship with God less about fitting in at church and more about discovering the Man behind the testimonies.

It was the wisest thing I ever did. I became so convinced of God's grace, love, and strategy for us all, that I wanted to tell every person I could. At first this was through a blog, then a book. Eventually I communicated my message through speaking, and from there it evolved into a movement. I decided the only way to convince a generation about God's grace was to be honest about my mistakes. I bore my truth.

This honesty helped others feel seen and awakened their hunger to trust God for more than their fears. Still, when I held the Book that reflects God's heart the most, I could not find a woman to whom I could relate. Sure, Sarah didn't believe in God when He promised she would receive a child, but that wasn't the same as a general disbelief in God.

Then I found her. She, like Dr. Anita, caught me by surprise. Yet there she was, clear as day, as if she'd come to accept that her story would be overlooked for those of other, more virtuous women. The first woman created—the one who was deceived by a serpent and ate from a tree. The woman who questioned whether she could trust God and whose name bears the shame for causing humanity's fall is the woman who held up a mirror that finally made me feel seen in Scripture.

Eve's life became a lesson in scars and grace that deepened my faith that God is with us even in our worst mistakes. I intently studied the few verses we have about her story. I looked at her life from every possible angle and even founded a movement that centers on the revelations I discovered. At first I thought the serpent initiated his attack by getting inside Eve's head, but he couldn't get in her head until he first broke her heart.

In Genesis 3:3–4 the serpent says just enough to make Eve distrust God's intentions for her life and the directions He left behind. Yeah, Eve is my sister because heartbreak is what did it for me too. It wasn't that I didn't fit in at church. It wasn't that I wasn't good enough to experience the love of God. It wasn't that I was too lost ever to be found again. It was the heartbreak that my eight-year-old self experienced that robbed me of my power.

The early stages of my ministry taught me that God could use broken hearts. However, in the last few years I've learned that God wants to mend those hearts more than He wants to use them. I would have settled for the honor of just being used, but there was an undeniable dissonance between the beauty unfolding in my life and my ability to embrace it fully.

Have you ever been so excited to hear your favorite song that you didn't care that your speaker was broken? Sure, there's a buzzing hum like a symphony accompanying your favorite music, but the song is too good to turn off, so you ignore the buzz and sing along. That's what it felt like living out God's restoration in my life.

If I were a faulty speaker humming in the middle of the church, someone would disconnect me from power so the service could continue. But this was a hum that no one could hear but me. I was still showing up for work. I was still volunteering, cooking, cleaning, and showing up for my family, but there was a humming underneath it all.

Then, similar to how Eve appeared on my radar out of nowhere, Dr. Anita Phillips entered my life. She'd been around, but I hadn't taken the time to connect with her. It took only one encounter to realize that the women I served could benefit from her brilliance. I asked her to join me in helping women clinging to hope when faced with seemingly impossible circumstances. The humming in my life was none of her business.

Our focus was supposed to be on others. I wanted to create an atmosphere where women could practice vulnerability and transparency. I desired nothing more than for every modern-day Eve to finally feel loved, valued, and seen regardless of their choices, history, or memories. I needed Dr. Anita to help us confront the shattered pieces of our hearts. I prayed that every woman could have a moment when they returned to their personal garden of Eden and began to heal.

It didn't take long to realize that I was attempting to lead where I'd never been. I needed to be guided by Dr. Anita more than I needed to partner with her. That hum was her business after all. She did not just take us back to the moment when life upended our faith and confidence. She took us to the garden within.

Silence falls like a weighted blanket over a crowd of thousands. Then, like a gardener putting on their gloves to pull weeds, aerate the soil, and water seeds, Dr. Anita puts her research, knowledge, and experience into a glove of wisdom and compassion. Suddenly, under the sound of her voice, every heart comes out of hiding and surrenders to overdue tending.

Dr. Anita's work is delicate enough to ensure the heart is not further damaged but precise enough to remove the weeds while maintaining the harvest. She speaks the words that have been stifled and releases the peace that has been waiting to bloom. The aftereffect hits their eyes before they even open their mouths. A brightness returns. A power lifts their head higher. An awakening has taken place, and their influence has been restored.

I will never tire of seeing Dr. Anita's genius at work. Whether in our late-night text exchanges or before a crowd of tens of thousands, she has an uncanny ability to help you realize that the more willing you are to embrace your humanity, the more powerful you can become. Not long after being under her tutelage, my relationship with God deepened.

The more I understood my emotions, the more specific my prayers became and the closer I got to God. I stopped hiding from His presence when I was overwhelmed, and instead I began running to Him armed with my truth. I thought I couldn't connect with God, but in reality I couldn't connect with myself, so I had very little to give Him.

It would not be hyperbole to say that Dr. Phillips has changed my life. I could take up the entirety of this book speaking of her brilliance, achievements, and accolades, but the evidence of her intelligence will be undeniable with a one-page turn. So I'll leave you with what I believe is the most impressive feature of her qualifications. She is not a coach who has never played the game. She's not a surgeon who has never experienced the lacerations of a scalpel. You're not just reading a book from a world-renowned thought leader in mental health and faith. You're receiving the truth from someone who knows this journey too well.

Her words are not laced with self-righteousness, nor do they condemn. She doesn't care how long ago you were wounded or how many times you've repeated the same thing. Instead, the words in this book have been marinated with compassion, coated in wisdom, and warmed with love. My friend, Dr. Anita, has already considered how cautious you may be to dive into the sea of emotions you think will overwhelm you. She'll be gentle. She'll be honest. She'll be loving because she takes the honor of tending to your heart seriously.

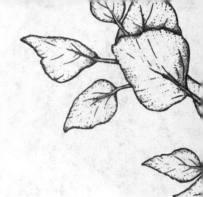

THE SECRET THAT JESUS KNEW

> God knew what he was doing from the very
> beginning. . . . The Son stands first in the line of
> humanity he restored. We see the original and
> intended shape of our lives there in him.
> ROMANS 8:29 THE MESSAGE

In 2022, I traveled to eight cities in two weeks. I met thirty thousand people and almost all of them were in the same kind of pain. I was part of a bus tour. For those of you who have not yet had the opportunity to have a bus-tour experience, that means twelve people shelved on stacked bunks, speeding down dark highways, falling asleep in one city and waking up in another. I loved every minute. And no, I wasn't trying to avert a midlife crisis by joining a band before my body's clock struck fifty. I was traveling and ministering with a women's empowerment movement called Woman Evolve. It's led by Pastor Sarah Jakes Roberts and that year we were on The Revolution Tour.

Every night in every city, thousands of people were invited to set an intention for their own personal revolution. Pastor Sarah asked them,

"What do you want to overthrow?" Every night in every city, they named a common foe.

- "Insecurity."
- "Grief."
- "Anxiety."
- "Fear."

No matter the name, the enemy was the same: their emotions.

Emotions are consistently cast as the opposition in a war that never seems to end. The scorched earth of your heart bears the scars, but your heart was never meant to be a battlefield. Your heart is a garden. I wish I had known that about my own heart sooner. I wish I had learned the strength, beauty, and importance of my emotions as a child, or as a young adult, or at least by the time I was a new mother. Like a lot of people, I grew up believing that I was meant to harness the power of my mind to live well and that emotions were nice but more often problematic. I spent decades ignoring that part of myself. Maybe you did too. Maybe you still are.

For some, battling emotional pain is a visceral reality. You and your feelings in hand-to-hand combat every day. Up close. Personal. Bloody. Others have perfected the sniper approach. You've built a sturdy wall around your heart and now spend most of your waking hours perched on top, scanning for anyone or anything posing a threat: disappointment, rejection, confusion, fear, or overwhelm. Opportunities for love or joy may even be eliminated if they never seem to last anyway. Of course, there is a third option: let the pain in and hold it prisoner. In doing so, you acknowledge emotion's immense strength, but, unable to wield greater power, you settle for a cheap substitute: control. Eventually, after those feelings have been locked away for so long, you forget they're even there. You embrace an induced amnesia for the sake of a previously unattainable peace. But that peace is precarious. An unholy earthquake will eventually shake the foundation of your life. Those prison doors *will* swing open, and then the battle resumes. The piercing sadness from that breakup is back. The resentment from that betrayal returns. The fear of failure runs wilder (and stronger) than ever.

None of these approaches to "managing" our emotions really work, do they? So why do we keep fighting? Power. War is always about power. We don't like to acknowledge the strength of our emotions because it seems like an admission of defeat. This may be *especially* true if you are a person of faith, and (can I keep it real?) it seems like, no matter how hard you try, your faith isn't leading you to green pastures and still waters the way it looks like it's doing for other people. If any of this sounds even remotely like you or someone you love—and you're wondering if there is another way—this book is for you.

Grappling

If you ask anyone who knew me growing up whether they are surprised to hear that I wrote a book about embracing emotion, I believe they would all say, "Yes! Absolutely shocked!" I have always loved books, data, and a well-thought-out argument. I'm embarrassed to say this now, but there were plenty of times in my life that I was grateful I wasn't as "emotional" as some other people I knew. I liked being the cool, calm, collected one who figured things out. I decided to study human behavior precisely because I wanted to figure some things out. I imagined that one day I would write a book about trauma or mental illness. In these pages we will talk about both, but this book is about so much more. You never know where life will take you. Let me tell you how I got here.

I am a trauma therapist. Most people end up in my line of work because of their own trauma. I am no exception. If you have seen me speak in person, you might have heard this when I was introduced: "Dr. Anita was raised in a family that grappled with mental illness." *Grappled.* Such a tidy word. But living it was messy. I grew up in a religious family. My maternal grandfather founded two churches. As I pen these words my father has been a senior pastor for nearly fifty years, and my mom has been a traveling evangelist for almost as long.

My parents' beliefs were in no way confined to the church building. At home, whether washing dishes or vacuuming, Mommy was almost always "praying in the Spirit." You could always find a bottle of anointing oil under the kitchen sink. There were basement prayer meetings. And only gospel music was allowed. We went to doctors and hospitals when we were sick, but we were also told that prayer could heal. We were taught to believe in the protection of angels. We learned about demons, too, and scriptures to disrupt their work. As a child, I saw miraculous things happen. I never doubted our faith, so when a demon showed up in the doorway of the bedroom I shared with my older sister Valerie, I thought I knew what to do. I didn't see it, but she did.

The first time her demon appeared, Valerie's terrified screams snatched me awake in the middle of the night.

"What, Val? What? Why are you screaming?" Her eyes were wide open, so I knew it wasn't a nightmare.

"There's a demon at the door, 'Nita! There's a demon at the door!"

I glanced over there. The door was open, and the hallway was dark. "Val, I don't see anything."

Her screams were too loud for her to hear me. I knew Val's cries would soon wake my parents and they would come to help us, but each scream cut me like a razor blade. I couldn't take it anymore. Shaking with fear, I whispered a prayer of protection and ran through that doorway to go get my dad. He was already in the hallway running in our direction. Dad didn't see the demon either, so he wrapped his arms tight around my sister and started praying. My mom was behind him, standing with me. We prayed too. Val squeezed her eyes shut and the screams gradually subsided. Finally, she opened one eye to peek. The demon in the doorway was gone, but not for good.

That awful scene happened over and over. Valerie was about eleven years old then. I was only six. Her screams became my midnight alarm clock. I started getting anxious. It became hard for me to fall asleep. A few years later, when our room became my room, at bedtime the first thing I did was close that door. Although I never saw it myself, Valerie's demon had become my demon too. I would be twenty-eight years old before I could fall asleep in a room with the door open.

As an adult, my sister was diagnosed with schizophrenia, a mental illness that sometimes includes seeing and hearing things that aren't there. Today, those who have this illness can live well with ongoing treatment, but Valerie was born in 1969. Back then, it wasn't about my religious parents refusing to believe in mental illness. There was simply no real mental health conversation in our community in 1969. Or 1979. Or 1989, for that matter. I host a faith and mental health podcast called *In the Light*. My mother was my first guest. During that talk with her I learned that Valerie's earliest symptoms emerged when she was around five years old. Looking back, we can see it, but at the time, our family had no idea what was happening.

My sister was tormented by the sight of that demon for close to a year, and then it stopped. We didn't know it then, but Valerie had been exposed to illegal drugs and realized they kept the hallucinations away. Freedom from that torment was too much for any child to resist. By her late teens, Val was addicted. Drug use led to her spending much of her life in the streets, but when she was about forty years old, she went to the last of many addiction recovery programs and was finally able to stop using. She strengthened her relationship with Jesus. She got treatment for her mental illness. She got a good husband. She got a whole lot of joy. And then she got to see God face-to-face. Her body bore the destruction of the years her addiction stole. She was almost fifty when her heart stopped beating. My sister didn't die by suicide, but I still consider untreated mental illness her cause of death.

Valerie did once receive professional mental health care as a young person. A crisis during her sophomore year in high school led to four months at a psychiatric hospital. It did not go well. The professionals assigned to her, and the culture of the institution, felt incredibly foreign (and at times condescending) to my family, both as people of faith and as African Americans. The staff there either didn't know how or didn't care to bridge the divide between their world and ours. So I became one of them. I became a mental health professional, but there were questions my training alone could not answer.

"I Still Want to See It in My Bible"

I once heard my mom say, "I know something is wrong and that Valerie needs more help than we can give her, but I still want to see it in my Bible. How can I understand it in my Bible?" I was just a teenager then, but I made a silent promise to find the answer to her question.

Conversations at the intersection of faith and mental health have been contentious for a long time, and in many ways they still are, but I see progress. The overwhelming impact of what began in 2020—the Covid-19 pandemic; vicious debates about closed churches, masks, and politics; heightened experiences of racial trauma and injustice—seemed to inspire a truce between faith communities and the mental health community, albeit an uneasy one. The emotional suffering wrought by the pandemic wasn't choosy. People of all faiths or no faith found themselves newly in the grip of depression, anxiety, panic attacks, and addiction relapses. More churches than ever began discussing mental health from their platforms, in their staff meetings, and online with their parishioners. It was encouraging.

But I call the truce *uneasy* because it was born of necessity rather than resolution. A lot of questions that bolstered and sustained that divide persist, and for many practicing Christians, my mother's question remains: How can I understand it in my Bible?

My mother's question was so powerful because it wasn't an either-or question. It was an everything question. It was a big-picture question. My parents taught me to look for God everywhere and in all things. They encouraged my work and my research to help prevent the type of pain our family endured with only one caveat: never choose an answer that limits God.

Over the years I carried my mother's question with me. The shape of the question changed but the essence remained the same. It began as "How do we understand mental illness through the Bible?" but evolved into "How do we understand wellness?" Is well-being simply the absence of pain? If it's more, then where should all these healing journeys lead and how will we know when we get there? What was the Creator's original intent when humanity was formed? *How does Scripture define* well-being?

I waited a long time for that answer only to find out it has everything to do with our hearts. I can't wait to show you how Scripture clarifies again and again that it is the heart—not the mind—that God designed to be at the very center of the human experience, and that *includes* our feelings. I believe this book will change the way you think about how you feel. But, just in case you are reluctant to join me on this journey because you believe that "emotional" is mutually exclusive with "powerful," let's wrap this introduction by turning our attention to Jesus.

Jesus, His Emotions, and His Powerful Life

Jesus stood in front of Lazarus's tomb and wept (John 11:35). When He showed up in Jerusalem and found the temple set up to change money instead of lives, Jesus unleashed a whip and table flips (Matt. 21:12). Later, in a garden, wrestling with the most intense feelings of anguish we can imagine, our soon-to-be Savior turned His face toward heaven and begged to be rescued from a brutal end (Luke 22:42). Then on the cross, about to offer His last full measure of devotion, Jesus hit the hardest wall of all—He couldn't feel His Father's presence. Jesus expressed those feelings of abandonment, distress, and despair through the words of Psalm 22:1. He asked a question that pain would one day plant in my heart and in yours. Jesus asked His Father *why* (Mark 15:34).

Jesus literally knows what our hearts feel in our weakest moments because He felt it too. How do I know? Because the Bible tells me so.

> For we have not an high priest which cannot be touched with the feeling of our infirmities; but was in all points tempted like as we are, yet without sin. (Heb. 4:15)

This verse tells us that Jesus experienced every form of physical *and* emotional pain that we do. Not only that, but Jesus also expressed those feelings with His words and through His body—which means feeling isn't failing because Jesus never failed.

Have you ever deeply grieved the loss of a loved one and then felt guilty for not feeling better sooner since you know that you will see them again in heaven? Have you ever been rightfully furious but held it in because you believed it would be wrong to express your anger? Have you ever felt like a faith failure because fear tied your stomach into knots? Have you ever desperately wanted an explanation from God but thought you might be struck by lightning for crying out, "Why?"

If having and expressing those feelings wasn't a sin for Jesus, then it's not a sin for you. No emotion is a sin.

Let that sink in.

Now ask yourself whether you have ever berated yourself for feeling something that Jesus felt too. We spend so much time and energy fighting a part of us that brings us closer to being like Him. That revelation alone is worth the price of admission—but there's more.

- After Jesus wept at Lazarus's tomb, He raised Lazarus from the dead (John 11:43–44).
- After Jesus demanded order at the temple, He performed healing miracles (Matt. 21:14).
- After Jesus endured Gethsemane's agony, hundreds of soldiers were knocked to the ground by the power of His words alone (John 18:6).

- After Jesus absorbed the sear of separation at Calvary, His decision to die shook the ground, tore a thirty-foot temple veil in half from top to bottom, and set the stage for victory over death itself (Matt. 27:51–52).

In each of these instances we see Jesus' pained heart give way to a supernatural display. Jesus knew the secret of the connection between our hearts and a powerful life. It's time for you to know it too.

So I'm going to say to you what I said to those thirty thousand hearts that gathered for The Revolution Tour in 2022. You don't need to overthrow your emotions to experience a revolution in your life. You just need to overthrow the lies you have believed about your emotions. The Creator designed your heart to be a garden, not a war zone. A truly powerful life isn't won. It's cultivated. This book will take you on that journey.

In part 1 you will discover how nurturing your emotional well-being positions you to unleash spiritual power. In part 2 you will discover how your emotional life waters the garden of your mind. In part 3 you will discover how emotional health nourishes your physical health—and strengthens your embodied garden.

Are you ready to end the war with your emotions and embrace the powerful life you were created for? If so, the first step is easy: turn the page.

Part 1

SOIL POWER

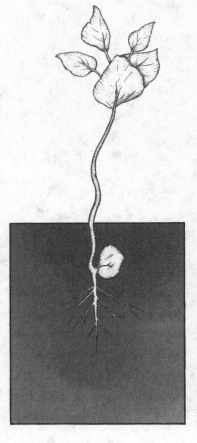

Throughout history, people of many religions have sought spiritual insight amongst seeds, soil, plants, and fruit. Seeking those insights through the lens of my own childhood faith, I learned that gardens are more than a metaphor. The soil of our hearts nourishes our lives spiritually, mentally, and physically. I invite you to walk the garden with me. Together we will discover how important our emotions are to living a powerful life. For part 1 of this book, we will focus on spirit and address these questions: What is the heart-spirit relationship? How does our emotional health influence our spiritual health? How can heart-work unlock spiritual power? The answers are in the garden.

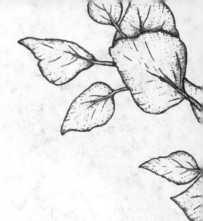

Chapter 1

THE SEEDLING

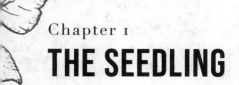

> Thou shalt be like a watered garden.
>
> ISAIAH 58:11

For nearly two weeks I left early every morning. Rushing the whole way, I covered the three blocks between my house and my middle school in record time.

My inspiration? Pea plants.

On the morning that our fifth-grade science teacher announced that we would grow our own pea plants, I had glanced around, looking for bags of soil, but there weren't any. I raised my hand.

"Mr. Rhodes, where's the dirt?"

He smiled. "When we plant seeds, it can take quite a while to see a sprout. A lot has already happened by then, even though we didn't see it. This experiment will help us understand how plants grow by letting us see what happens underground." My ten-year-old heart was instantly aflutter—he had me at "understand." I love knowing the why and how of things.

Mr. Rhodes had each of us fill a clear plastic cup with wet paper towels instead of dirt. Then, we wedged our seeds between the paper towels and the sides of the cup so that we could watch them grow. We checked on our seeds every day, but a few minutes of observation at the beginning

3

of class couldn't possibly satiate me. I had to get there early to stare intently at each new development in my own cup and everyone else's. The root piercing the seed's hard shell. The sprout meandering upward. Something usually hidden was being revealed, and I didn't want to miss a thing.

By the time the experiment ended, the seed had disappeared. A tiny plant had taken its place. I carried my seedling to our house, dug a hole in our vegetable garden, and covered its fragile roots with soil. Although my pea plant now had a real home, I missed spending the extra time with my science teacher. I loved spending time with all my teachers. School was always my safe place. My teachers saw that I was a bright and curious student. What they didn't see was that beneath the surface, some painful beliefs had already taken root in my young heart. It would be years before anyone could see what was growing, but a lot was already happening underground. Looking back, I think that's why I was so attached to that seedling. She was so vulnerable. I wanted to protect her the way I wished I could protect myself.

The Soil of Our Hearts

A child's heart is rich soil. The younger they are, the more fertile that soil is. Almost any seed planted there will grow. By the time I was writing down middle school science observations, the sexually abusive experience that I kept secret from my parents had already planted a destructive belief in my saddened heart: *I am different.* When after always trying to be a good girl I was still harshly punished for a simple mistake, fear awakened a new belief. I scribbled that seed's name in my lock-and-key diary: *People only love you when you're good.* When the chaos wreaked by my older sister's mental illness consumed my family, frustration allowed this seed: *I am on my own.* That is not to say that no good seeds were planted. There were plenty. After my first Easter Sunday speech, the congregation's applause and my father's proud expression watered my heart with joy and *I am a good speaker* took root. When my mother smiled despite her tears, looked me in the eye, and said, "No matter what we go through, it's not God's fault. He will help us understand it," assurance filled my heart: *God has the answers.*

As I got older, my heart remained fertile ground for all those seeds; they reproduced well into my adulthood. I continue to nurture the good ones and have embraced the hard work of breaking unhealthy cycles. However, I do admit there is one stubborn weed that constantly reappears. It's called *perfectionism.* Perhaps you have seen that one in your garden. If not, I'm sure you have your own painful weeds to pull. Lots of different things grow in the same garden. My pea sprout did not supplant my dad's tomatoes and collard greens; it grew alongside them. Joy doesn't negate pain and pain doesn't negate joy. Real life happens in the both-and zone.

I never forgot my pea plant, but if you are wondering whether she inspired me to become an avid gardener, the answer is no. I don't have a green thumb. Bugs disturb me deeply and I've never met an earthworm I liked. That said, my sprout wasn't finished with me yet. Twenty-three years later she would lead me to a garden I had spent my life searching for even though I didn't know it. It was there that I discovered the answer to my mom's question.

The Discovery

In 2007, I found myself in science class again. This time, I was studying the brain instead of plants (or so I thought). That curious fifth-grade girl was now a wife, a mother of two young children, a minister, a licensed therapist, and a PhD student. The class wasn't required for my degree, but despite the chaos of my busy life, I felt so strongly drawn to the course that I sacrificed my summer break to enroll. As the class began, I was also starting a deep dive into the book of Romans. That "book" is actually a letter that's included in the New Testament, written by the apostle Paul to the first-century church in Rome. It contains some of the most controversial passages in the entire Bible. Never one to shy away from hard topics, I was eager to study it for myself, but I barely made it through the first chapter before being arrested by this verse: "For since the creation of the world [God's] invisible attributes are clearly seen, being understood by the things that are made, even His eternal power and Godhead, so that they are without excuse" (Rom. 1:20 NKJV).

I was stunned. In all my preacher's-kid life, I couldn't remember a sermon centered on that verse—and believe me when I say that by thirty-four years old, I had heard a lot of sermons. Questions filled my mind: *Creating the heavens and the earth wasn't just God preparing a fabulous place for Adam and Eve to live? I can understand things about who God is by studying the things that God made?*

Have you ever had a moment you knew would change things forever? Maybe it was the first time you stepped onto your college campus, or when you got the job offer, or first laid eyes on the person you would eventually marry, or held your new baby in your arms. Whatever it was, you knew nothing would be the same again. For me, that scripture on that day was one of those moments.

My study of Romans took a detour straight to the first chapter of the book of Genesis. I wanted to read the story of creation with fresh eyes. What had I been missing? I scoured the emergence of the heavens and the earth with rapt attention to every detail. A deep knowing was springing up within me. I believed I was meant to discover something important in my neuroscience class, so I prayed, "God, You led me to take this course. You created this world, and You created our bodies. As I study what You made, help me to clearly see and understand something new about You. Amen." Our prayers don't always get answered right away, but this one did!

The next day my class reading assignment introduced neurons. Your body is made up of trillions of cells and there are hundreds of different kinds. A *neuron* is one kind of cell, and you have billions of them. Their job is to send and receive information. It takes thousands of neurons working together to form just one of the seventy thousand thoughts we have every day.[1]

When I saw a drawing of a neuron for the first time, it caught me off guard. It looked so familiar—my pea plant! There it was. I couldn't help but laugh with surprise. That neuron looked like a seedling. I jumped on the internet to search for more pictures of neurons and found one that looked like the illustration in my textbook. Then I searched for a picture of a seedling. I placed the pictures side by side and stared and stared, and stared some more. Why? I was looking directly at two things God made, and those two things looked alike. Scriptures began to float to the surface of my heart, verses and passages that used flourishing gardens to describe human flourishing.

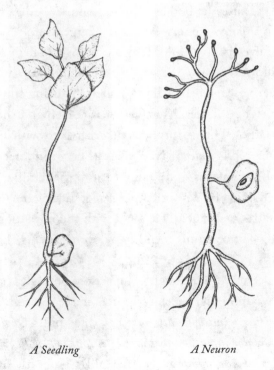

A Seedling   *A Neuron*

Psalm 1:3 says that we "shall be like a tree planted by the rivers of water," and in Jeremiah 32:41 God says, "I will plant them in this land." I remembered that Proverbs 11:28 tells us that "the righteous shall flourish as a branch." And there are so many more. One of my favorites is Isaiah 58:11: "The LORD shall guide thee continually . . . and thou shalt be like a watered garden." In an instant my worlds collided. Theology, psychology, and biology were all suddenly in the exact same place—and that place was a garden.

The Choice

I'm not really a sci-fi fan, but *The Matrix* is one of my all-time favorite movies. The main character, Neo, is a young computer programmer who has no idea that his life isn't real. Earth has been captured by diabolical machines that use the bodies of living human beings for fuel. The machines hide this by keeping everyone plugged into a virtual reality program. The lives people think they are living are happening only in their minds. However, there is a group of revolutionaries who know the truth. They have escaped the Matrix and are battling the machines to free humanity. Their leader, Morpheus, visits Neo and shows him life outside the Matrix. Then Morpheus presents Neo with two pills and one choice: One pill is blue. If Neo takes it, he will forget the truth he just saw with his own eyes so he can return to the familiar, albeit false, reality he's been living in. The other pill is red. Taking the red pill means leaving the Matrix permanently to fight with the revolutionaries and to experience a revolution in his own life by overthrowing the lies he had believed.[2]

This may seem like a dramatic comparison, but that's how that neuron and that seedling and those scriptures made me feel. *Do I chalk it up as an interesting coincidence and move on* (blue pill)? *Or do I act on the belief that the Creator intentionally shaped neurons to look like plants to teach us something about how He made us* (red pill)? Honestly, it was a very intimidating choice. I was a student in a PhD program in counseling at a Christian university where we were being taught that the Bible's revelations were limited to religious topics like sin, salvation, and eternal life. It was not intended to answer psychology's theoretical questions, and biology was definitely not included. I knew pursuing this parallel could lead to my work being rejected—as both a misuse of Scripture and an invalid source of knowledge for psychology.

There was an outside threat too. I was a serious student hoping to ultimately pursue public health research. It's one thing to study spirituality generally as a path to meaning and connection. It's a whole other thing to start applying spiritual information to neurons! I would risk being dismissed by the academic and professional communities I so wanted to be a part of. But I was staring at a neuron—the basic building block of the mind—alongside Scripture and a plant. *What might I find out if I choose to believe that I really am seeing a God-thing?* Then my mother's voice reminded me: "Never choose an answer that limits God."

I chose the red pill. And I am still choosing it because I am continually overwhelmed by the mysteries the Creator has been unveiling ever since. In the counseling room, at church, and in my own life, these lessons have resulted in a lot of insight and a lot of healing. But I can imagine just seeing and hearing it now, for the first time, it might seem a bit "out there."

More Than a Metaphor

Plant and garden metaphors are built into the way we speak. In American English, we have phrases like:

"I liked the city, so I put down roots."

"If you see a problem, nip it in the bud!"

"Make sure you don't miss the forest for the trees."

We use garden metaphors every day without even noticing. I think that makes it easy for us to see that language in Scripture without thinking much about it. The Bible consistently uses plants and gardens to teach critical spiritual lessons and general principles for living. Now we see there's a deeper reason for that. The similarities between neurons and plants challenge us to broaden our view of God and our expectations for this sacred text.

Metaphors often use two unrelated things to clarify how we feel. When an exasperated mom says, "This room is a pigsty!" she is saying that the disgust she would feel standing in a pigsty is similar to the way she now feels standing in her teenager's bedroom. Metaphors can teach us about feelings. Pause for a moment and consider how you feel about the thoughts that drive you crazy. You probably feel emotions like frustration, exasperation, or despair. But what if I said, "A thought is a plant"? How does that invite you to feel differently? A plant is something to be nurtured. We heal a struggling plant by giving it the care it needs, right? What if you responded to painful thoughts as evidence that something within you needed to be nurtured or cared for? That's how metaphors change feelings.

But this plant-neuron connection is more than a metaphor.

Another teaching tool that uses comparison is called an *analogy*. An analogy is like a metaphor in that it compares two unrelated things, but instead of teaching us how things *feel*, analogies teach us how things *work*. For example, after discovering the relationship between an atom's nucleus and its electrons, chemist Ernest Rutherford explained it by saying that electrons orbit the nucleus the way planets orbit the sun.[3] We don't need a chemistry degree to understand what Rutherford was saying. Analogies use a familiar thing to teach us about a new thing. But this plant-neuron connection is more than analogy too!

The similarities between plants and neurons go beyond appearance. There's a functional similarity as well. Like plants in a garden, the neurons in our bodies are very close to one another but not directly connected. There is a tiny space between each of them. When your leg itches, neurons work together to tell your brain to tell your hand to scratch that itch! To accomplish this communication, one neuron releases a chemical that carries the message across the space to the next neuron, across a vast chain of neurons, until that itch gets scratched.

Plants communicate with nearby plants the same way. For example, if a plant's leaves are touched by the leaf of a neighboring plant, it can send a chemical message through its roots and across the soil space to the roots of nearby plants to let them know that things are getting crowded. The plants respond by changing their growth pattern.[4] Plants and neurons look alike, *and* they act alike. And there is more. Some things are actually the *same*.

Consider this: the chemicals our neurons use to send messages are called *neurotransmitters*. Guess what? Plants use some of the *same* chemicals, including neurotransmitters known to affect our moods (dopamine and serotonin), fuel our stress response (norepinephrine), activate our muscles (acetylcholine), and help our bodies rest (melatonin).[5]

What I saw in that neuroscience class all those years ago revealed a relationship beyond anything I had ever considered possible. Neurons come in many shapes. Some look like a blade of grass. Others look like a bush, a meandering vine, or a tree. But all of them look like plants, and God planted billions of them all throughout our bodies.

The Creator gave us gardens to teach us about Him and about how He designed us in His image. You have just had your first glimpse of a beautiful and awe-inspiring reality. The Creator planted a garden *for* us, and then the Creator planted a garden *within* us.

> The Creator planted a garden *for* us, and then the Creator planted a garden *within* us.

The Parable

There at my kitchen table, in the middle of a perfectly regular homework assignment, on what had begun as a perfectly regular day, the answer I had long been seeking was found hiding in plain sight. How does Scripture define *well-being*? As a garden. That's the answer.

Having found this neuron-garden, I was ready to discover all sorts of spiritual insights about the mind, but Sister Pea Plant kept me from getting ahead of myself. She had another bit of wisdom to share. I remembered gingerly burying her roots in our family's garden. My pea plant would not survive and grow to fulfill her pea-producing purpose in the plastic cup I got from my science teacher. Her life depended on where she was planted.

A garden is more than plants. It begins with seeds and eventually produces fruit, but it's the soil that holds it all together. A flourishing garden depends on good soil. So how does this apply to us? If plants represent our thoughts, what do seeds teach us about? What does fruit teach us? And most importantly, where is the garden planted? *What does the ground represent?*

In chapter 13 of the gospel of Matthew, Jesus tells us a story called the parable of the sower. In that story, a gardener scattered seeds freely even though he knew that there were different kinds of soil in different parts of the field. The seeds ended up on four types of ground; three of the types presented pretty serious growth challenges.

Some of the seeds landed along the edges of a well-worn path. Jesus described those seeds as having fallen by the *wayside*. Nothing could grow there because the ground was hard and dry. It couldn't absorb the seed. Those seeds were vulnerable; birds ate them (v. 4).

Another area of the field had *stony* soil. There, the seeds found enough water to come alive—but not enough to *stay* alive. The plant grew tall quickly, only to be scorched by the hot sun (vv. 5–6).

That field also had a *thorny* zone. That soil nurtured the seed, and a plant began to grow. Its fruit was developing nicely at first, but it was choked by thornbushes before the fruit could ripen (v. 7).

There was *good ground* in the field too. The soil in those zones unleashed the full potential of all the seeds. Some yielded a thirtyfold return, some sixtyfold, and some even gave the gardener a hundredfold return (v. 8).

Every element of the garden is accounted for in this story and, when Jesus interprets the parable, every element of our inner workings is revealed. Jesus tells us that the seeds are words. The fruit represents what we do. What does the ground represent? Our hearts (vv. 18–23).

Your heart is the soil where spiritual seeds are planted.

Your heart anchors the roots of your mind.

Your heart nourishes the fruit you produce.

Your heart is the soil of your life.

While I didn't recall having ever heard a sermon preached about that verse in Paul's letter to the Romans, I had heard plenty of sermons about gardens. But none of them prepared me for what gardens teach us about well-being and the life our Creator designed us for. From the garden of Eden, to the garden parables, the garden of Gethsemane, the Garden Tomb, and the Garden City, the narrative is consistent.[6] A garden's condition depends on its soil; the condition of the garden within you—spiritually, mentally, and physically—depends on the soil of your heart. That means embracing your feelings. All of them. And that means it's time to end the war.

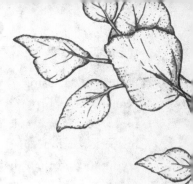

Chapter 2

CHECK THE FLOW

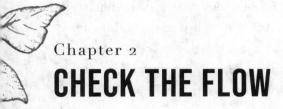

> Keep your heart with all vigilance, for
> from it flow the springs of life.
> PROVERBS 4:23 ESV

I peeked down at my phone and saw a new text message:

> "Dr. A., I have a friend whose little girl died in a house fire. She is searching for a trauma therapist, so I thought of you. Her name is Maria. She's a powerful woman who just needs some help right now."

It would be hard to find anyone who would *not* have described Maria Colón-Johnson as powerful.[1] The fire that killed her daughter was intentionally set. An eighth grader who lived next door had been brought to the attention of the police and social services after setting a fire in the supply closet at his junior high school. Standing there in the school office, the boy's father had assured them all that his son's obsession with science had just gotten the better of him. Not wanting to see a "good kid" get tangled up in the juvenile justice system, they let his dad take him home.

That summer, the family enrolled their son in a chemistry camp and even converted their backyard shed into a makeshift lab for him. Six months later, using a trail of accelerants ordered online, that thirteen-year-old boy purposely set six connected row houses on fire during the night. Maria was able to carry her young son out of the house, but her husband, Jerome, had collapsed, unconscious from smoke inhalation, trying to find their daughter, who had left her bed to sleep in the fairy-princess fort she had built in her bedroom closet. First responders were able to resuscitate Jerome but not their beautiful daughter, Gracie. She was one of more than a dozen people who died in the fires. Many others were injured, including several first responders.

Despite her trauma, Maria remained a devoted mother to her surviving child and had recently celebrated him receiving a full scholarship to college. She had completed the MBA she was working on at the time of the fire and was now running a foundation to fund research and develop policy initiatives to eradicate racial disparities in the juvenile justice system. Maria was a frequent speaker on national news outlets and had written award-winning think pieces for some of the most respected publications in the United States. She was also a staunch advocate for the right to grieve in a world that desperately wants the bereaved to "move on."

No one would say that Maria Colón-Johnson was not a powerful woman—except for Maria Colón-Johnson. She had done many things we would *call* powerful, but Maria rarely *felt* powerful. And she was tired of being described as "strong." After the parent of another child killed in the same fire died by suicide, Maria knew it was time to seek help.

In one of our early sessions, she said, "Everyone wants me wearing a T-shirt with #BLESSED printed on it. I hate it so much. It makes me feel like I'm falling short of Christian victory or something. Yes, it's been eight years and yes, my daughter being killed is still shredding me inside. They tell me God will give me beauty for ashes, but I don't believe that. Maybe beauty *with* the ashes, but how can an exchange happen? They say, 'God will give you double for your trouble' like He did for Job, but there is no replacing my daughter's life. It's not possible."

I responded by saying nothing. We sat in silence, allowing her pain to take up all the space it was due. A tear escaped Maria's left eye. Narrowly evading her effort to wipe it away, that tear slid down her cheek and fell on her blouse. And then another. And then another.

"This is the first time I have cried in front of another person since my daughter's funeral," Maria said. I didn't say it at the time, but I knew that first tear was her first step to living a truly powerful life.

Casualty of War

When I first met Maria, her heart was far more battlefield than garden. She was a casualty of the emotion war in two ways. First, while she was acutely aware of the constant dull ache of her grief, Maria was committed to keeping her painful emotions locked away for fear the pain would "win." She was also afraid that her grief and sadness would be too much for other people to handle. That's the second way that Maria was being wounded by this war.

Prevailing attitudes toward emotion, especially emotional pain, cause many people to struggle not only to be present with their own feelings but also to resist minimizing someone else's pain by encouraging them to be optimistic, think positive thoughts, or remember to be grateful. Those things are certainly good for us, but if the real goal is avoidance rather than growth, that kind of positivity becomes toxic. Pain denied is pain multiplied. It will only continue to undermine our well-being, and if we refuse to engage long enough, our spiritual health will decline.

Your spiritual life cannot be isolated from your emotional reality. Just as the soil can determine the fate of a seed, your heart can determine the state of your spirit. Scripture affirms this.

> And they came, every one whose heart stirred him up, and every one whom his spirit made willing. (Ex. 35:21)

17

> The boldest heart will melt with fear . . . every spirit will faint. (Ezek. 21:7 NLT)

> My servants shall sing for joy of heart, but ye shall cry for sorrow of heart . . . and vexation of spirit. (Isa. 65:14)

> A merry heart maketh a cheerful countenance: but by sorrow of the heart the spirit is broken. (Prov. 15:13)

In those verses, feelings of desire, fear, joy, and sorrow *preceded* a spirit that was willing, faint, full of praise, or broken. Proverbs 15:13 affirms that this heart-spirit connection is more than coincidence. The verse says that the spirit is broken *by* sorrow. Our hearts influence our spiritual well-being in a way that has nothing to do with sin. That is why, when Maria voiced her anger about the verses offered to comfort her (Isa. 61:3 and Job 42:10), I didn't hear a lack of faith. I heard her broken heart. Why strive to repair a broken spirit without caring for the sorrow that crushed it in the first place? Her feelings didn't need to be ignored. The soil of her heart needed to be watered.

So how did this war begin? Why do we believe the negative things we believe about emotion? We'll dig deeper into the garden shortly, but first we need to answer that question.

Why Do We Feel the Way We Feel About How We Feel?

When I started graduate school back in the late nineties, I didn't realize how old, wrong, or pervasive our destructive view of emotions was. But reflecting now, I recognize it in how I was being trained as a therapist. Emotions were seen as symptoms. Obstacles. Like an unruly child to be managed or a lion to be tamed. Until that first neuron led me to the garden within, it hadn't occurred to me to wonder what the Creator had intended for us in the beginning. How did we get here? The answer may surprise you. The roots of this modern perspective are very old.

A seed was planted by a Greek philosopher named Plato (428–347 BC). He described the human soul as driving a chariot pulled by two competing horses. One horse was more honorable and obedient. The other horse represented irrational passions. The rational mind drives the chariot. It must control the horses to achieve its goals.[2] While neither horse was perfect, Plato viewed feelings negatively (except for compassion and *platonic* love). "He regarded the emotions as irrational reactions of the lower psychosomatic levels of the soul."[3]

Plato's division between thinking and feeling became a defining feature of Western culture: mind good, emotions bad.[4] It caught on big-time, and centuries later we still see the fruit all around us. We see it in decades' worth of scientific research motivated to understand the brain and keep emotions at bay. We see it in a kid rushing to the school bathroom so no one will see them "crying like a baby." It's a client telling me what they *think* even though I asked them how they *feel*. It's a scientist's easy embrace of a theory that says the rational brain is more evolved than the emotional brain.[5] It's also a minister saying that God doesn't care about how you feel—He's just waiting for you to renew your mind.

Christians often pride themselves on having a biblical worldview, but that distinction is more easily claimed than lived. Plato died hundreds of years before Jesus was born, yet his ideas affected Christianity in a way that is likely hurting your life. Plato's disdain for emotion influenced another philosophy called Stoicism. The goal of Stoic therapy was to root out and destroy emotion. Blending the work of Plato and the Stoics, early theologians argued for freedom from emotion as a goal of *Christian* perfection.[6] And still today, so many Christians feel they are failing for feeling.

I grew up immersed in the best traditions of the African American church, where the cultural view of emotion was, in some ways, different from the mainstream Western perspective. Historically, in the Black

19

church emotions are felt, seen, and heard. From the preaching style to the physicality of worship to the shedding of unrestrained tears at the altar, we do emotion with our whole bodies. With that said, there is an even greater emphasis placed on a mental strength that is defined by not allowing our feelings to influence our decision-making or lessen our endurance. We are allowed to feel emotional pain, but it's a "shed your tears, then stand strong" type of thing. You can even skip the tears if you like, but mental strength? Nonnegotiable.

All religious traditions are influenced by culture. Your faith community may have taught you similar lessons or you might hail from spaces with different views. Maybe sermons at your family's church were meant to evoke peace and calm rather than shouts of victory. Perhaps it was fine to express happiness, but too much emotional pain was frowned upon. Maybe prolonged sadness or anxiety was seen as evidence of a hidden sin or simply irrelevant to the spiritual task at hand. No matter where we come from, one thing seems to be consistent: church messages about emotion often sound more like the world we live in than the Bible we are supposed to live by (Mark 7:7; Rom. 1:22).

What Would Jesus Do?

We're a long way from the WWJD (What Would Jesus Do?) days of the 1990s, but it's still a good question, especially when it comes to how we feel about our feelings. In the introduction to this book, we saw the example Jesus set for us through His own emotional experiences. In Scripture, we see Jesus authentically and *publicly* expressing His feelings. When I first explored emotion as a theme in Jesus' life and realized that His most emotionally intense expressions were closely followed by moments of undeniable power, I was as stunned as anyone. When we describe similar moments in our own lives, it's usually couched in the language of failure.

"I tried so hard not to cry, but I finally broke down."

"I was doing okay, and then I just lost it."

Why do we say things like that? What broke? What did we lose? And is that what you would say about Jesus at the tomb of Lazarus, or in Gethsemane, or on the cross? Did Jesus finally just lose control? Did Jesus have a breakdown? Considering the miracles displayed in the aftermath of Jesus' emotional moments, ask yourself this: Was Jesus breaking down or was He breaking through?

But Dr. Anita, you might be thinking, *Jesus is God!* Yes, He is. But Romans 8:3 says that once Jesus agreed to leave heaven, He received a human body. Being the fully divine Son of God didn't protect Jesus from having a fully human experience. When we resist leaning into Jesus' humanity, we devalue the depth of His sacrifice and underestimate the breadth of His love.

Jesus is our standard for Christian perfection. He is our example for walking out this human experience we call life, and He never condemned Himself for feeling. Jesus never once said, "I rebuke this sadness!" or "I rebuke this anger!" or "Get behind me, emotions!" Never once. Jesus was real about where He was and how He was feeling. In prayer, Jesus cried out to His Father *honestly*. Genuinely. Authentically. If you have ever tried to calm down or gather yourself emotionally *before* you started praying so that you could come to God the "right way," it's time to say no to Plato and the ways that culture distorts our view of our hearts.

Disconnecting from your feelings is not an act of faith; it's an act of avoidance. The unresolved pain is still there, beneath the surface, eroding your well-being. It is only our *unattended* sadness, anger, and fear that eventually threaten the ground of our hearts, not the feeling itself. We can absolutely stand on God's Word while equally making room for authentic emotional expression and healing. Your emotional pain is not mutually exclusive with your spiritual power. Jesus showed us that.

> **Your emotional pain is not mutually exclusive with your spiritual power. Jesus showed us that.**

A Love Story

I never get tired of talking about the heart. My passion is renewed by every person who finds freedom from the war they have been waging within themselves against themselves. Old habits die hard, so keep reminding yourself that emotional disconnection is *not* a spiritual discipline. Emotion is an active ingredient in your spiritual life, so the wise move is to take good care of your heart. That good care begins by seeing your heart the way that God does.

Your heart is important to God. Nearly every living thing on earth depends on soil to survive because plants grow there and, one way or another, plants feed nearly every living thing.[7] The Creator of the heavens and the earth knows all about soil, so we should pay attention to what that means. Your heart is the soil of your whole life too. That tells you how much your emotional well-being matters. Scripture places the heart at the very center of the human experience.[8] The Bible attributes the entire spectrum of emotion to the heart.[9] Our hearts are capable of being gentle or arrogant, loyal or deceptive, pure or perverse. Either way, the Bible identifies the heart as defining who we genuinely and authentically are—the real us (Prov. 27:19).

Your heart is immeasurably valuable to God. That includes your feelings.[10] From Genesis to Revelation, the gospel is revealed through a love story about a seed and its soil. That soil means so much to Jesus that He called Himself *a seed* (John 12:23–25). When the garden of Eden was created, Jesus was there. John 1:1 says that Jesus was the Word the Creator spoke when the heavens and the earth were made. When Adam and Eve stumbled into a harsh new world, the Word went with them as a seed embedded in the embodied garden of a woman, traveling down through generations until the day of His birth (Gen 3:15). Wrapped in a living, breathing, flesh-and-bones body, the Word-Seed stepped into our world to love us in person. Then Jesus died so that He could one day grow as a tree of life within us, planted by the rivers of our hearts. The heart-spirit relationship is the story of soil and the seed it was made for.

The soil is the love interest in this true tale. That's how God feels about your heart. That's how I want you to feel about your heart. That's how I want you to feel about *you*.

In parts two and three of this book, we will look at how cutting-edge science is catching up with what the Bible has long said about our hearts, but first I want you to step into the garden to learn what the Creator has been trying to teach us about emotion all along. If your life is anchored in Scripture, I hope that you are already being transformed simply because you trust the pages of this sacred text and the depths of the wonders it holds, even when—*especially* when—it surprises you.

The Heart-Spirit Relationship

In the parable of the sower the seeds are words (Matt. 13:19). Seeds teach us how the words we hear become the truth we believe. Jesus, the living Word-Seed, wants to be planted in your heart because that's where belief begins (Mark 11:23; Acts 8:37; Rom. 10:9).

A seed is a living plant in a dormant state. The seed waiting to release the tiny plant tucked inside of it doesn't need to be planted to come to life. A seed is not dead; it is only sleeping. When the seed awakens, things start moving in the soil. The seed pulls air and water from the ground into itself, swelling larger and larger until it breaks open. That moment is called *germination*. In your heart, the moment a word-seed germinates is called *belief*. The gospel of Luke explains it this way: What?! A seed doesn't have to die in order for the planted to grow.

> Now the parable is this: The seed is the word of God. Those by the way side are they that hear; then cometh the devil, and taketh away the word out of their hearts, *lest they should believe* and be saved. They on the rock are they, which, when they hear, receive the word with joy; and these have no root, *which for a while believe*, and in time of temptation fall away. (8:11–13, emphasis added)

This passage shows us that belief requires a seed-soil match. That's why we don't believe everything that we hear. If the soil doesn't possess what the seed requires, it remains dormant. If the soil has even the bare minimum of the required qualities, the seed awakens, but its full potential remains unrealized. The plant dies. In the soil of a fertile heart, those words will awaken and unleash their *full power* to bear abundant fruit in your life. A seed needs only two things to wake itself up: air and water. That's why my pea plant was able to germinate tucked within the folds of a wet paper towel in a plastic cup; it had air and it had water. But a seed's natural habitat is soil, not a paper towel. Good ground is fertile. Fertile soil allows air and water to flow through it. In the garden within, air and water are about *faith* and *feelings*.

Faith

A belief is different from a fact.

Mr. Walt Disney opened his first theme park in 1955. That is a fact. Liberian Nobel Laureate Ellen Johnson Sirleaf was the first democratically elected president of an African nation. That is a fact. Facts are visible, measurable, and objectively verifiable. A *belief* is the "acceptance of the truth, reality, or validity of something . . . in the absence of substantiation."[11] That evidence gap is the difference between a fact and a belief. Facts don't require faith. Beliefs do.

A seed needs air to germinate. In the soil of your heart, faith is air. Faith makes room for the seed. Then, when a word-seed awakens, faith flows through your heart into the seed, but faith is not an emotion. Faith is not a thought either. Faith is spirit. It's breath. Genesis 2:7 says that when God formed humanity His breath brought us to life. It became our *neshamah*, which refers to both the breath of God and the human spirit.[12] Remember, a belief is something we accept as true even though it can't be substantiated by our five senses. Faith substantiates. Faith bridges the evidence gap by saying "Yes!" to the possibilities that a word offers you. Faith opens our hearts to believe.

Feelings

If you are a follower of Jesus, His word-seeds should be falling on your heart often, not just on the day the relationship began. If they are, then you know that those seeds can land in different places on different days. I am always fertile ground for, "Take delight in the LORD, and he will give you the desires of your heart" (Ps. 37:4 NIV), but Jesus' words about forgiving people "seventy times seven" times (Matt. 18:22) have required me to tend to my stony patches on seventy times seven occasions. We can have absolute faith that the words of Scripture are true and powerful, but where we are emotionally can influence whether God's Word awakens within us.

Water's significance for literal gardens teaches us about the role of emotion in the garden within. In the parable of the sower, Jesus uses emotions to describe how the soil types are different. Wayside soil is hard and dry—no water. The stony soil starts out joyful—there was enough water for the seed to awaken, but when the heat came, joy evaporated and anger remained. There was enough water in the thorny soil zone, too, so Jesus' word-seed came to life—but so did the thorny weed of anxiety. Sometimes we feel more than one thing at the same time. The relationship between water and emotion is more than a metaphor—there's a biological manifestation too.

Intense emotions often draw water from our eyes. Sometimes there is sadness in our tears. We may even cry until it seems there is no water left, and we feel dry and numb. At weddings and graduations our eye-water has joy in it. And tears aren't the only water that flows with our feelings. We sweat in response to both giddy excitement and crippling fear. Even the water in our mouths flows with our feelings. Because anxiety directs our bodies to send more water to our sweat glands, it makes our mouths dry. Empathy affects the water too. A research study published by Austrian scientists in 2021 asked participants to watch a film that inspired feelings of empathy. Researchers took samples of participants' saliva before and after the film to assess the presence of emotion- and stress-related biomarkers. Empathy affected the chemical composition of the samples; it influenced what was *in* the water.[13] When it comes to our emotions, there is definitely something *in* the water!

Dry ground can never be good ground. It is impossible for soil to be fertile without water. When a seed awakens, the water flows in until the seed literally bursts. The living plant that had been tightly contained inside is freed to grow. There is something special about that life-awakening flow. We call it *hope*.

> Faith says, "It's possible." Hope says, "It's possible *for me*."

Hope is the *feeling* of expectation. Faith says, "It's possible." Hope says, "It's possible *for me*." Hope is what possibility feels like. Hope is the basis for every other pleasurable emotion we experience. We can't experience feelings like joy and peace when we are hopeless. Hope is a catalyst. It moves us from word-seed to the fruit of action. Hope hydrates us for the sometimes arduous journey of growing into all that we were created to be. Hope motivates. *Motive*, *motivation*, and *emotion* all share the same Latin root word: *movere*. It means "to move."[14] That movement begins in the heart. And it begins with the flow of hope.

Let It Flow

Words are full of creative power. Your heart is the ground where word-seeds are planted. They are not sown in your mind. They are sown in your heart—the same place that your feelings live. That was the Creator's design.

All words are seeds. God's words are the most powerful seeds of all, but our words have power too. That's why we should be careful about how we speak to others and to ourselves (Job 26:4; Prov. 18:21; Eph. 4:29). Word-seeds can become beliefs.

Our beliefs are formed by both faith and feelings. That's important because our beliefs about God, our identity, our relationships, and our purpose determine our spiritual well-being. How we are doing emotionally can, and usually does, influence how we are doing spiritually. That's a big deal.

Does that mean every painful emotion is spiritually dangerous and we should avoid feeling them at all costs? No.

Does that mean that Jesus was sometimes dry or stony or thorny ground? Also no.

How do we reconcile this? The answer is, when it comes to how we are feeling, we need to let it flow.

A well-watered garden is in a constant state of flow. Too much water leaves no room for air. The seed suffocates and drowns. Too little water and those word-seeds remain dormant. Likewise, the beliefs that inform our spiritual well-being are nourished by both faith and feelings. When we resist our feelings, we risk undermining the soil's fertility in the long-term. It's best to do what Jesus did: allow the flow. When my heart is dry, tears of joy water me. When my heart is overwhelmed, tears of sorrow are drainage.

That's why I said that Maria's lone tear was the first step to living her most powerful life. She finally allowed some drainage. In the months that followed, Maria's broken heart continued to heal in new ways. In the safety of our time together, she became more and more comfortable acknowledging and expressing her emotions. Maria finally felt as powerful on the inside as she had been appearing on the outside. She began living from the heart, not in spite of it.

Is Maria's grief gone once and for all? Of course not. Does she still get angry? Absolutely. But now she allows the pain to flow through her and out of her. That made space for more joy. And that healing flowed into her spiritual life.

A little more than a year into our work, Maria was using session time to reflect on some great things she had experienced in the previous week and how much her hard work in therapy had changed her life. She smiled and said, "You know, I think I'm starting to understand what 'double for your trouble' might mean. Nothing can ever replace my daughter, but I am glimpsing new possibilities."

"Wait a minute!" I replied. "Are you saying you are ready for a T-shirt with #BLESSED on the front?"

"I think I might be!" Maria laughed—and that laugh was some of the sweetest fruit I ever tasted.

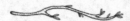

The first step to living a powerful life is to commit to cultivating a state of emotional well-being that will catalyze, sustain, and nourish what we choose to plant. Emotional well-being does not mean that we are always happy. Emotional well-being is our capacity—and willingness—to feel all our feelings. It requires us to be aware of, acknowledge, and experience our feelings. In fertile soil the moisture levels fluctuate. What's *in* the water fluctuates. Fluctuation is not the problem. Stagnation is.

Being emotionally well isn't about earning something from God. Your emotional well-being won't affect how God shows up for you, but it might affect how you show up for God. When we are emotionally healthy, we position ourselves to be more powerful spiritually. That is why, for me, being a therapist is a divine calling. *Your heart is a sacred seedbed*. Emotional healing is sacred work.

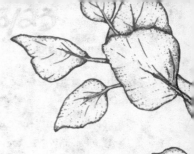

Chapter 3

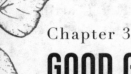

GOOD GROUND AND YOUR MOST POWERFUL LIFE

> God called the dry land Earth . . .
> and God saw that it was good.
>
> GENESIS 1:10

I placed my lunch on the faculty lounge table and slid into the seat across from my coworker Casey. He didn't have his usual upbeat energy that day, so I wanted to check on him.

"Hey, Casey, you seem a little down today. I'm happy to be a distraction, listen, or leave you alone if you need space. What might help the most?" *Give choice.*

Casey exhaled audibly. "I really appreciate that," he said. "I would love to get out of my head and talk. My thirty-fourth birthday is coming up. I know it's not that old, but I feel like time is catching up with me and I haven't accomplished everything I should."

I waited for him to gather his next thought. He soon continued.

"Lately I've been feeling God wants me to move on with some big goals, but I've been too hung up on the 'how.' Every year when my birthday arrives, I go into reflection mode. I evaluate the year and if I don't feel like I've progressed enough, I start feeling down. I feel like I'm not really becoming the person I need to be."

Casey's words went straight to my heart. I know what it's like to wonder if I'm *not* doing something I should be doing to live out God's will for my life. We can really paralyze ourselves with that, so I hoped to encourage my friend.

"Casey, sometimes we 'become' as we go. In 2 Corinthians 4:7, we're reminded that we 'have this treasure in earthen vessels.' We are clay pots—both strong and fragile—so we go forward knowing it's not us but rather God in us. Maybe instead of waiting until your next birthday to look *back*, it might help to try looking *forward*. Maybe set some very achievable goals for this coming year, and then let God put His extra on it? And if you would like to share those goals with me, I'd be happy to be excited about them with you!"

Casey's face brightened. "I love accountability! Once I jot them down, I'll share."

A couple of weeks later Casey sent his goal list:

1. Get my idea for a business networking platform off the ground.
2. Create more passive income.
3. Become more whole (more connected with myself and God).
4. Lose fifty pounds; get healthier.
5. Travel more, including seeing my family throughout the year.
6. Finish building out my home music studio.
7. Make more music.
8. Be more present in my marriage (stronger, healthier marriage).

Casey had clarity about what he wanted to accomplish, which was great. But I remembered him mentioning feeling down about not having made the progress he wanted in the previous year, so I guessed that a few of the items on his list (maybe more than a few) had been goals for some time. He needed a new way of looking at his life.

Working up the courage to try again can be tough, especially when we feel like we have failed before. Sometimes a perspective change breathes fresh life into our efforts, so I took the risk of reorganizing Casey's list and emailed it back to him. Here's what it looked like now:

- Relationships
  - With God and with myself
    * Become more whole (more connected with myself and God).
    * Take better care of my body (lose fifty pounds; get healthier).
  - With my family
    * Be more present in my marriage (stronger, healthier marriage).
    * Travel more (including seeing my family throughout the year).
- Purpose
  - Get my idea for a business networking platform off the ground.
  - Make more music.
- Legacy
  - Create more passive income.
  - Finish building out my home music studio.

"Hey there!" I wrote. "I organized your goals into three 'life zones': relationships, purpose, and legacy. Those are the three dimensions of a powerful life, and I believe you'll find it helpful."

Casey wrote back the next day: "This is amazing and so helpful! The outline really unpacked my goals and laid them out in a way that's easier to digest."

When we met up in the faculty lunchroom a couple of weeks later, Casey was still feeling inspired. "I really enjoyed thinking about my life in terms of relationships, purpose, and legacy. Those categories cover what I want to accomplish, but they also capture how I want my life to feel. Where did you come up with these?"

"Well," I replied, "I found them in a garden."

Joanna's Lemon Tree

A lemon tree planted in the shadow of Mount Tamalpais taught me about the three life zones: relationships, purpose, and legacy. I'd gone to Mount Tamalpais to refill my heart. I had been tired for weeks and extra sleep wasn't helping. I was irritable, struggling to concentrate, and nagged by a headache. Those are all signs of emotional exhaustion, so when I got the chance to spend a few weeks alone, off-grid, I didn't hesitate. I rented a room in a quaint one-hundred-year-old house owned by a lovely couple named Rob and Joanna who were enjoying their golden years. And the best thing about this place was the lovingly curated garden that surrounded it.

When Joanna gave me a tour of her vibrant, lush garden, I was immediately drawn to the lemon tree. As soon as I laid eyes on it, my body wanted to collapse in its shade. Somehow, the lemon tree spoke to my weary heart, offering rest and peace through its shady foliage and beautiful fruit.

One morning early in my stay, I found Joanna at the kitchen table reading her Bible. She offered me a seat, cool water in a mason jar, and warm lemon crumble breakfast cake. Joanna was elated to find out that I did ministry work and asked if she could pray for me. I barely exhaled a yes before crying. Oh, how I needed that. Joanna prayed over me almost every morning of my stay, and each time another piece of me came back to life. I had gone there to sleep and to breathe, but God had so much more in store.

During one of our many conversations, I asked Joanna to tell me about the lemon tree. She told me that California is the best place in the United States to grow lemon trees because the soil there is like the soil in Italy. It has everything that lemon trees need.

I had never considered the soil as a factor for where a citrus tree might grow. If (in some random game of Trivial Pursuit) I had been asked what lemon trees need, I would have said warmth and lots of sun. And lemon trees do need those *external* things, but every tree begins as a buried seed. Until Joanna told me how much the soil mattered, I had taken its contribution for granted, but as with most things—including us—what's happening on the outside is secondary to what's happening on the inside.

You know by now that if something sparks my interest, I am going to research it, and that's exactly what I did. Curiosity led me to an old study by the University of California Wildland Research Center.[1] The researchers wanted to test the soil in the area, but the thick overgrowth prevented them from taking soil samples directly. Instead, they flew over the wildlands, taking photos, and then classified the soil that they couldn't see, based on plants that they *could* see. They divided the area into *life zones* based on what was growing there. For example, one life zone had mostly grass while another life zone only had small bushes.[2] You never know where spiritual insight is waiting for you. Those life zones got me thinking about the parable of the sower.

When I teach about wayside soil, stony ground, thorny ground, and good ground, people immediately start thinking about what might be *wrong* in their lives.

"Am I stony ground?"

"I'm thorny ground for sure!"

And then, "How do I fix it?" I get it. I am always scanning my own heart for issues, and anytime we encounter God's Word it's natural to seek an opportunity to be better, but let's be careful about always seeing ourselves through the lens of insufficiency.

In his book *The Pastor*, Eugene Peterson said this:

> People . . . are defined by their creation in the image of God, living souls, whether they know it or not. They are not problems to be fixed, but mysteries to be honored and revered.[3]

I love that Pastor Peterson saw his congregants that way. I see my clients that way. I see my family and my friends that way. I see you that way. How do you see you?

I think it's wonderful that we live in a time when people are so aware of the importance of healing, but we are more than the sum of our broken parts. So before we dig into healing the rough patches in your heart, let's explore the good ground that Jesus mentioned (Matt. 13:8). Like the soil in the California wildlands, we can take a snapshot of your garden within and identify good ground based on what's growing there. *But Dr. Anita, the parable only tells us that good ground gave an abundant harvest. The Bible doesn't tell us what was growing there.* I beg to differ.

Eden, Life Zones, and Growing Your Most Powerful Life

On the first day of creation, obscured by darkness, our planet lay hidden within the waters like a baby in the womb waiting to be born. On the third day, the Creator broke the waters, and the ground came forth. The waters were called *seas*, and God saw that the water was good. The ground was called *earth*, and God saw that the ground was *good ground*. On that day, the Creator went out to sow. Word-seeds fell on good ground for the first time.

> And God said, Let the earth bring forth grass, the herb yielding seed, and the fruit tree yielding fruit after his kind, whose seed is in itself, upon the earth. (Gen. 1:11)

That ground was fertile. Three types of plants grew. What can we learn about the powerful life we were designed for based on what the Creator chose to plant? Since there were three types, let's imagine a garden with three life zones: the first life zone for where grass grew (relationships), a second life zone for herb-yielding seed (purpose), and the third life zone for fruit trees (legacy). Grab your journal—this Eden exploration will also be our first official tour of your garden within.

The Relationship Zone

The Creator planted grass first. I believe that grass teaches us about relationships. Grass is the plant-sonification of "the more the merrier"—it's all about togetherness. While each blade may be the individual product of a single seed, when does anyone ever plant *one* grass seed? Never. A single blade of grass does not a pasture make. We are created to thrive in relationship with God, and with others. All of that begins within you.

Your relationship with yourself.

A healthy relationship with yourself requires self-awareness, self-love, and self-care.

Self-awareness includes:

- Being aware of and connected to your body.
- Knowing how you feel, what you need, and what you want.
- Recognizing your thinking patterns, character traits, and strengths.
- Acknowledging your weaknesses.
- Being accountable when your behavior doesn't align with your values.

Self-love says things like:

- I am worthy of being loved, valued, treasured, and respected.
- My voice matters.
- I will treat myself with kindness, even when I let myself down.
- I am both imperfect and capable of growth.
- I don't mind if other people see my imperfections.

Self-care includes intentionally choosing to nurture yourself spiritually, emotionally, mentally, and physically, not after but before your breaking point.

Your relationship with others.

Relationships are our most powerful, and most overlooked, self-care tool. When we nurture our relationships, they nurture the ground of our

> **When we nurture our relationships, they nurture the ground of our hearts in return.**

hearts in return. Grass roots are thin and widespread—perfect for keeping vulnerable soil from falling apart. And because those grass blades are so close together, they protect the soil on the surface too. How do you know if the grass in your garden is thick and thriving? Here are some things to expect in healthy relationships:

- You want to share your good and bad news.
- You feel supported and loved.
- You feel safe enough to be completely you.
- You don't mind asking or being asked for help.
- You accept others, invest in them, and love them unconditionally.
- They feel the same way about you and want to do the same for you.

For many people, marriage and family provide these close relationships. Marriage can be a wonderful experience, but too often we emphasize it to the exclusion of the power of friendship. Friendship matters too. A lot.

Your relationship with God.

I used to lead an eight-week relationship seminar. Participants completed a questionnaire rating various aspects of their lives. One question was, "On a scale of 1 to 10, how strong is your relationship with God?" No one ever gave a 10/10 rating, and everyone described improvement in terms of *doing* more. "Pray more." "Go to church more." "Read my Bible more." Our spiritual disciplines are very important, but *doing* isn't all there is. Like any personal relationship, our relationship with God includes an emotional connection.

Your relationship with your Creator is unique because you are unique, so I can't offer you an exact way to measure it. But here are some questions to evaluate the relationship for yourself.

Do you feel with the holy Spirit or watched by them only?

GOOD GROUND AND YOUR MOST POWERFUL LIFE

You are God's child (1 John 3:1). In a healthy parent-child relationship we grow up with a sense of safety, consistency, and unconditional love. The child trusts their parent. Our relationship with our own mother and father can shape this dimension of our connection to God. How do you feel about the idea of God as a parent? Have you experienced safety there? Is there anger or confusion? How have your life experiences shaped this divine relationship?

Jesus calls you friend (John 15:15). Look again at the list of things we expect in a healthy relationship. Those are the ingredients of a great friendship! How do you feel about the idea of Jesus as your friend? Have you experienced support and unconditional love there? Do you cry, laugh, and share your feelings? How have your life experiences shaped this divine relationship?

The Holy Spirit lives within you (John 14:26). The Holy Spirit comforts us and advocates for us from _within_ us. That's a deeply personal, deeply vulnerable relationship to be in. How do you feel about that type of intimacy? Are you consistently aware of the Spirit's presence within you? When you are aware of it, does it feel like being _with_ or being _watched_? How have your life experiences shaped this divine relationship?

Four of Casey's goals were in the relationship zone. I especially love the way he worded this one: "Become more whole (more connected with myself and God)." Casey instinctively recognized that our relationship with ourselves and our relationship with God are inseparable. As you reflect on those questions about your own relationship with the Creator, I'm sure you recognize it too!

How's it growing in your relationship zone?

Before we move on to discuss the next two life zones we find in Genesis 1, let's pause to consider your personal relationships. Where is the grass greenest? What's going well in your

37

relationship with yourself? Which relationships with others hold your heart together on hard days? Which dimension of your relationship with God do you lean into most? Wherever you are thriving in your relationship zone, you just found good ground!

The Purpose Zone

After grass, the next set of plants that good ground brought forth was seed-bearing plants. Like you and me, seed-bearing plants weren't created just to exist for existence's sake. God attached purpose to these plants. We were created to live with purpose too.

For some people, just talking about their purpose is stressful. The intense pressure we feel to find and fulfill *the* purpose we were created for (lest we completely fail at life) is our own invention, not God's. Purpose is not "the thing you are supposed to do." Purpose, simply defined, is a reason *why*. We are meant to live intentionally. To move with a why. To live *on* purpose. Seed-bearing plants teach us three things about living on purpose garden-style.

First, *purpose meets a need*. Our Creator gave us these plants for food (Gen. 1:29). Think of them as crops. Wheat is a great example of this kind of plant because it is used to make bread. Food is a fundamental need. Seed-bearing plants were provided to sustain us. We, too, should seek to meet needs that sustain others. In seeking to live on purpose ask yourself, "What need(s) do I desire to meet?"

Second, *purpose is productive*. These crops are working plants. They have a *goal*: to multiply by making new seeds. They are all about productivity! But these plants weren't all the same. The Creator expected them to be productive "according to their various kinds" (Gen. 1:11–12 NIV). We are working plants, too, called to be productive according to our various kinds of gifts. Those gifts are the mechanisms by which we can meet needs. Proverbs 18:16 says, "A person's gift makes room for him and brings him before great people" (NASB). Great people can help you meet more needs! That's the goal, right? To live on purpose ask yourself, "What gift(s) do I have to offer?"

One of the problems with defining purpose as "What *I* am meant to do" is that it breeds self-focus. The third thing that seed-bearing plants teach us is that *purpose is relational.* It's about service. One wheat seed can become a stalk that produces a hundred new seeds. And that's just one stalk. That level of productivity isn't just for us. It's for those around us. Asking, "What is my purpose?" should not be synonymous with, "Who am I?" Let purpose ask, "What is my role *in my community*?"[4]

Your community relationships.

The life zones in your garden aren't divided by brick walls. A garden is an interconnected system where each part depends on every other part. Living on purpose depends on cultivating one more type of relationship: community. Whether it's our parents and siblings, the love of our life, or our most treasured friends, we tend to view all our closest interpersonal relationships as family, but we were also created to live in community.

Imagine standing on a lush lawn so big we would need a fleet of riding mowers to cut it. The greater the expanse of the grass, the more beautiful it is and the more we are in awe of it. That's how community is meant to feel. Some blades are so close together their roots touch. Others are separated by thousands of plants. Yet each blade nourishes and strengthens the whole. The same is true for us. We are integral parts of communities, filled with people we interact with every day and some whom we will never meet. Distance doesn't diminish the connection.

The life of Jesus makes this very clear. His purpose was fulfilled in community. Jesus chose to become one of us and then gave His life for all of us. Likewise, our individual decision to follow Christ is only individual for a moment. In the time it takes to say "Amen," we become members of a new community, the children of one Father "of whom the whole family in heaven and earth is named." With Christ dwelling in each of our hearts by faith, we are called to be *rooted and grounded together* (Eph. 3:14–17).

We are all members of many communities. Our neighborhood. Basketball fans. Everyone who graduated from our high school. Incest survivors. People who watch YouTube. Marathon runners. Single mothers. Refugees. Humanity—that one includes us all. There are so many communities that connect us. To live on purpose ask yourself, "Which of my communities am I serving?"

Like me, purpose might be infused with your job. My heart is deeply moved when people feel unsafe. We *need* safety. Teaching is my divine *gift*. In the community of *we* who have survived trauma, I teach others how trauma steals safety and how to heal.

We all *need* connection. That need deeply moves my son Michael's heart. People are easily comforted by his presence, so he made it a goal to *gift* comfort to the community of *we* who live in his Chicago neighborhood. Once on a visit, he took me to brunch at his favorite place. An older gentleman waiting tables there cried telling me how Michael gave him a birthday card that year. His why isn't connected to his remote tech job, but that is one of the several ways that my son is living on purpose. Purpose is always within reach.

How's it growing in your purpose zone?

Let's check on your crops. Living on purpose means having goals informed by a clear *why*. You can, and likely will, have more than one why at any given time. What *need* moves your heart? What *gift* have you offered to meet it? Which community— which *we*—have you served? Even if you have never thought of purpose this way before, I'm sure some beautiful work has already cropped up. Anywhere you are thriving in your purpose zone, you just found good ground!

The Legacy Zone

More than seventy years ago my father planted a pear tree in the front yard of the tiny cinder block house where he was raised. He is a great-grandfather now, and a fifth generation of our family will have the chance to rest in the tree's shade. Fruit trees were the third type of plant described on the third day of creation. These trees represent legacy.

Like the seed-bearing crops, fruit trees are also working plants, but the work of a tree takes much longer, and it lasts far longer. Crops like wheat live for only one season. At harvest time, the work is complete and the plant dies. In the same way, we can only live on purpose during the season that is our life on this earth.

Trees exemplify legacy because trees stand for generations. One of the oldest known trees is a Patagonia cypress located in Chile. It's estimated to be more than five thousand years old.[5] We can be sure that none of us will live that long, but we can all plant a legacy. Our legacy goals may be inspired by the same things that inspire purpose. The difference is legacy will far outlast us.

The idea of legacy is often connected with marriage and children. But that is not the only way to have generational impact, nor is it inherently a "holier" way. The apostle Paul never married, nor did he have children, yet his legacy is indisputable. Our definition of legacy is often too narrow, and we have done many unmarried sisters and brothers a disservice by emphasizing marriage and parenthood as the only or best way to leave a legacy. To quote Yana Jenay Conner, a favorite singles minister of mine, "If marriage and children was the pinnacle of the human experience, Jesus would have done it."[6]

Some pursue legacy by leaving a financial inheritance to community institutions and important causes. You can also leave a legacy by helping a family member with their college expenses, or writing down and sharing the lessons you have learned. Legacy is anything that leaves the world a better place. A retired pastor can mentor young ministers so that her hard-earned wisdom prevents them from burning out. A high school science teacher may dedicate himself to establishing science and

> Legacy work is all about love, pure and unconditional—pouring love into a future that we may not be present to enjoy.

technology programs in a historically marginalized community. Legacy work is all about love, pure and unconditional—pouring love into a future that we may not be present to enjoy.

How's it growing in your legacy zone?

Are there trees there? Even if it's one brand-new tree just starting to grow, it counts! Wherever you find one, you just found more good ground in your garden within.

Love: A Vital Nutrient

Let's pause for just a moment to take a closer look at love—because without this vital nutrient, the garden within simply cannot flourish.

You just identified the areas where your garden within is already thriving. Those areas of your life are powerful! Be it in the relationship, purpose, or legacy zone, we know that if those plants are flourishing, it's because you are breathing in the faith that says "It's possible!" and hope is keeping your heart watered. Fertile soil breathes. Fertile soil is well-watered. Fertile soil is also *nutrient-rich*.

All living things need nutrients to survive. We get most of our nutrients from food, but when you bite into that organic apple you found at the farmer's market, your first thought probably isn't, *Wow. Delicious. That farm must have amazing dirt*. But maybe it should be! Fertile soil supplies plants with as many as seventeen different nutrients. They dissolve into water and then flow into the plant. Those nutrients are directly connected to the strength of the plant and the healthy benefits the fruit

Love is the most important nutrient supplied
by the soil, through the water to the plant

offers. The same thing is true about us. Many things nourish our heart-soil, like joy, peace, and kindness, but *love is the most important nutrient*. Fruit nourished by love-rich soil is better in every way.

Dr. Robert Sternberg, a professor of psychology at Cornell University and a past president of the American Psychological Association, developed the Triangular Theory of Love. He defined love as having three components: intimacy, passion, and decision/commitment. Intimacy describes the feelings of close connection that bond us in relationship. Passion is about the drive that prioritizes that relationship. Finally, the decision/commitment component is about both the present choice to love right now and the determination to see that love last in the long-term.[7]

I like Sternberg's approach because I hear the echo of the garden. Love comes alongside the *faith* that connects us in all kinds of relationships (intimacy). It flows in with the water of *hope* that sustains us (passion), and then love strengthens us and nourishes us as we persist and complete the work (decision/commitment). When it comes to making sure our hearts are good ground for good things, remember this: "three things will last forever—faith, hope, and love—and the greatest of these is love" (1 Cor. 13:13 NLT).

Good Ground

So, there you have it, my friends. *How does Scripture define well-being?* As a garden.

What is meant to grow in that garden? Relationships, purpose, and legacy. These are the things that fill our lives with meaning.

Where is that garden planted? In the soil of our hearts.

What makes that soil fertile? Faith, hope, and love.

How do we keep the soil fertile? By cultivating emotional well-being.

What is emotional well-being? Our capacity—and willingness—to be aware of, acknowledge, and experience all our emotions.

What happens when we cultivate emotional well-being? We unleash, sustain, and nourish the full power of the word-seeds that we choose to plant in our garden within.

Is this what it means to live a powerful life? Yes.

Garden Goals

Think of someone you would describe as powerful. Why did you choose them? We usually call people powerful because of their effect on the world around them. Many have their names etched into the annals of history. Others are known only to our family, church, or community. Whether their achievements are linked to their social position, wealth, anointing, intellect, or charisma, we often make assumptions about what it must be like to be them. So we are shocked when a fashion icon dies by suicide and devastated when a power couple divorces. We are outraged when a moral leader turns out to be anything but, and relentlessly voyeuristic when our favorite singer checks in to rehab. Why? Because we believe if they achieved every goal on *our* list, they must have won the emotion war. But the heart wins every time, even when it's broken. Battling your heart is futile. Heal it instead.

Embracing life in the garden requires us to redefine what it means to be powerful. For Casey, that redefinition began by looking at his goals and then his whole life through Eden's lens. In the garden within, a truly powerful life isn't conquered. It's cultivated. In the garden we no longer idolize achieving *in spite of* our pain. We celebrate taking time to heal. When you live your life from the inside out—tending to your heart *first*—the life you produce will be a life you can sustain. And because healthy plants strengthen the soil in return, when I nurture my relationships, live on purpose, and grow a legacy of love, I produce a life that also sustains me. That is the most powerful life of all.

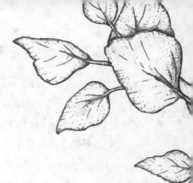

Chapter 4

GROUND ZERO

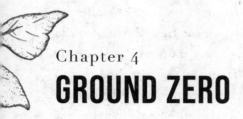

> Cursed is the ground . . . through painful toil you will eat
> food from it . . . . It will produce thorns and thistles for you.
>
> GENESIS 3:17–18 NIV

A couple of weeks after my coworker Casey and I talked about Eden's life zones, we met for lunch to make a plan that would increase his chance of achieving his goals that year. Casey hoped I would be one of the people in his life who helped hold him accountable to his plan. My answer was no. I told him, "Accountability isn't really my thing. But I am a great cheerleader!" Accountability can be useful but sometimes we use it inappropriately, as if the threat of being embarrassed for not having accomplished a goal on time will force us to achieve. I didn't want Casey to force his way forward. I wanted him to grow a sustainable life.

For example, let's say I decide I want a pear tree in my backyard. I buy pears from the grocery store, glue a string to each pear's stem, then go to my yard and hang the pears on a tree already growing there. Success! Well, sort of. I have a tree with pears on it, but I do not have a pear tree. A strong wind will confirm that. But this is the typical approach to achieving our goals: we wish them, we list them, and then we hop into Plato's chariot, determined to put "mind over matter" to accomplish those goals by any means necessary. Any means except getting in touch with the frustration, sadness, or fear that derailed us the last time, and maybe even the time before that.

Goals should not be gathered, they should be *grown*. Finding a way to get pears doesn't equate to having a pear tree. Caring for the garden within means moving from a conquest framework to a culti-vator framework—from the never-ending war to abundance. External motivators will take us only so far if our emotional well-being can't support the things we hope to grow. Forcing ourselves forward may yield a few successes, but we harm ourselves in the process. Instead of setting up external things to help you force your way to your goals, do a soil-check. Ask yourself, "What's going on *inside me* that's making this goal hard to reach?"

Goals should not be gathered, they should be *grown*.

Instead of promising accountability, I offered to do a quick soil-check with Casey, starting with his relationship goal to feel more connected to God.

"When you think about your relationship with God, what emotion comes up?" I asked. Casey looked confused. "What do you mean?"

I rephrased, "How do you *feel* in your relationship with God right now?"

Casey was silent for a while. He was so accustomed to jumping over or pushing past emotion to get something done that it never crossed his mind to consider his feelings. I asked him to take a few moments to imagine himself sitting in the presence of God. I let a little time pass and then asked, "What does it feel like to sit there?" He looked up and said, "I feel guilty."

Casey went on to share that he felt awful for not spending more time in prayer and when he did, he would wonder, *Am I doing this right?* He knows others who get up early and spend an hour in prayer, but when he tries that his mind wanders and twenty minutes in, he gives up. I recalled how Casey had said that he didn't feel like he was becoming the person he needed to be to do what God called him to do. I realized that Casey was concerned about not being good enough. That's not guilt, it's shame. An accountability partner and a dozen prayer-time alarm clocks weren't going to help with that. Casey wasn't failing for lack of willpower. He was stuck because of shame. That's where he was. So that's where we started. There was soil work to do.

I found relationship, purpose, and legacy in the garden of Eden, so I know they are essential to living a powerful life. The problem is we aren't in the garden of Eden anymore. The good and fertile ground that existed there has been altered, and we find that story in Genesis 3. The first two chapters of Genesis tell us how the garden of Eden came to be. The third tells us how that good beginning came to an end.

The End of the Beginning

On a certain day a serpent went out to sow. He was carrying a single word-seed to an exact location: the garden inside a woman inside a garden.

The Serpent found the woman exactly where he knew she would be—near Eden's forbidden tree. While the Creator had told the man and the woman not to eat fruit from the Tree of Knowledge of Good and Evil, the Serpent planned to get her to do exactly that. He surveyed her inner garden, found the most vulnerable spot, and carefully started digging a small hole in her heart.

> [The serpent] said to the woman, "Did God really say, 'You must not eat from any tree in the garden'?"
>
> "We may eat fruit from the trees in the garden, but God did say, 'You must not eat fruit from the tree that is in the middle of the garden, and you must not touch it, or you will die.'" (Gen. 3:1–3 NIV)

Affirming the Creator's words halted the Serpent's digging.

"You will not certainly die," the serpent said to the woman. "For God knows that when you eat from it your eyes will be opened, and you will be like God, knowing good and evil." (vv. 4–5 NIV)

This time she didn't respond, so her adversary was able to quickly resume his work; the hole in her heart-soil soon reached the perfect depth for the Serpent to plant his seed. As the woman turned her full attention to the forbidden tree, the Serpent silently planted its word-seed: *You can be like the Most High* (Isa. 14:12–14).

The possibility filled her like air flowing into her lungs. And, like water, a longing in her heart flowed in the same direction. The Serpent's word-seed swelled and broke open. The woman *believed*. Pondering the tree's most unique benefit—the elevation of her mind—clinched her decision. Then her husband made the same choice. They ate the fruit their Creator had forbidden. That was the end of the beginning.

We've Fallen and We Can't Get Up

Romans 5:12 says, "When Adam sinned, sin entered the world. Adam's sin brought death, so death spread to everyone" (NLT). Since everyone means everyone, we are all affected. In a sacrifice that will forever exceed my comprehension, Jesus was tortured and crucified to repair the damage Adam's choice created (Rom. 5:18), and His resurrection was a victory bequeathed to us. The Bible says that accepting Christ makes us a "new creation" (2 Cor. 5:17 NIV).

If you follow Jesus then, like me, you know how "new" showed up for you, but not *everything* was new, right? We still need to breathe, drink our water, and eat food. Some hard things stayed the same too. Even after deciding to follow Jesus, people can still catch colds, get sprained ankles, or develop an autoimmune disease. We know that the fall changed our bodies in a way that persists. But how does that translate to other things, like achieving the goals we glued to our vision board? How does what happened in the first garden help us understand today's struggle in the garden within? The answer is in the ground. It tells the story of how our whole lives became harder.

Adam and Eve (and that serpent!) each did something wrong, and each received specific consequences. But it didn't end there. Something also happened to the ground. Like you and me, the ground didn't participate that day, but after that, life in every zone was painfully different (Gen. 3:17–18).

The green expanse of grass withered away as the cursed ground dried and hardened. Now all relationships were harder.

Effortlessly abundant crops now struggled as sustenance demanded sweaty toil. Living on purpose was harder.

Flourishing fruit trees, ordained for generations, saw their fruit choked by thorny ground. Leaving a legacy was harder. As the soil transformed, the garden of God became a wilderness. Good ground is now ground zero. And it is there that Jesus takes us, to teach us about how the ground of our hearts changed. The parable of the sower takes place at the scene of the fall.

Ground Zero

Since the fall changed the ground, faith, hope, and love are no longer a given. Now sadness, anger, and fear are. This chapter digs into what the parable of the sower teaches us about those three emotions, and it uses three types of soil—the actual dirt outside of your house—to do it: clay, sand, and silt.

Sadness: The Wayside Soil

Jesus begins the parable with the seed that fell by the wayside and describes its loss (a bird eats it). At the wayside, we have gone from lush grass to this barren ground. From relationship to disconnection. Jesus doesn't attribute an emotion to this soil, but I believe that wayside soil reveals sadness.

Psalm 102:1 recounts "A Prayer of an Afflicted Person Who Has Grown Weak and Pours Out a Lament Before the LORD" (NIV). There the psalmist describes his own heart's journey from green pastures to the wayside:

> Hear my prayer, O LORD,
> And let my cry come to You. . . .
> *My heart is stricken and withered like grass,*
> So that I forget to eat my bread. . . .
> I am like a pelican of the wilderness;
> I am like an owl of the desert.
> I lie awake,
> And I am like a sparrow alone on the housetop.
> My enemies reproach me all day long . . . .
> Because of Your indignation and Your wrath;
> For You have lifted me up and cast me away.
> My days are like a shadow that lengthens,
> *And I wither away like grass.*
>
> (Ps. 102:1, 4, 6–8, 10–11 NKJV, emphasis added)

The psalmist is in relational despair. There are no friends spoken of, only enemies and the belief that God is displeased. The psalmist feels lonely, like a solitary bird. The sparrow on the roof is particularly poignant—sparrows like company, but this one is alone. Remember the seed that fell by the wayside? A bird ate it. Perhaps that lonely sparrow is the guilty party.

From *hurt* to *embarrassed* to *rejected* to *powerless*, sadness goes by many names, but we define it as "an emotional state of unhappiness, ranging in intensity from mild to extreme and usually aroused by the loss of something that is highly valued."[1] Disconnection is the essence of loss. A loved one dies. A friendship ends. A refugee misses their homeland. Each of these losses is a disconnection. When a business failure or a parent's rejection leaves someone trying to reconcile what's happened with who they *believed* they were, that's disconnection too.

The miry clay.

Clay is a type of soil that helps us understand sadness. It has two things in common with good ground. First, it's well-watered. It holds so much water that, just like sadness, clay is heavy—but water can be a good thing. Sadness, combined with hope, can inspire persistence and service in ways that reconnect us. Lots of water also makes clay nutrient-rich. In the same way, sadness can be rich with love. When we are sad, we are less judgmental, so we empathize more deeply with the pain of others. In that way, sadness strengthens life in the relationship zone.

The problem with clay is it has two extremes. The first extreme arises from slow flow. Clay doesn't drain well, so the water balance is easily thrown off. When there is too much water, clay gets sticky. Has sadness ever left you feeling stuck and desperate to be rescued? King David had that experience and was grateful to get out!

> He lifted me up from the pit of despair, out of the miry clay. (Ps. 40:2 BSB)

Because clay is so sticky, too much water eventually pushes all the air out. If we don't acknowledge and tend to our sadness, it may overwhelm us the same way. Breath is cut off; seeds drown. Heart translation? Faith fails; beliefs die.

> Therefore is my spirit overwhelmed within me; my heart within me is desolate. (Ps. 143:4)

To make sense of a profound loss, sadness can leave people questioning their beliefs, searching desperately in hope of finding an explanation. Hope unfulfilled eventually becomes hope lost.

And, as Proverbs 13:12 says, "Hope deferred makes the heart sick" (ESV). I believe a sick heart manifests as wayside soil.

Under incessant heat clay eventually dries out and hardens. When the water is gone hope is gone. In the same way, when our pain does not relent, hope can give way to powerlessness—a type of paralysis that leaves us feeling almost nothing at all. The road from sadness to hopelessness is usually a long one. Take care of your heart before it gets that far. "Just keep moving forward" doesn't always solve the problem.

Holding your breath.

Sadness can be a tough emotion, but at times it connects us in ways that help the relationship zone flourish. However, despair is an extreme that suffocates us. The longer we feel disconnected, the more likely we are to actually disconnect. We may abandon self-care, isolate from loved ones, and lose touch with our Creator.

For a Christian who wars with emotion by ignoring or minimizing their feelings, a crushed spirit may be the first time their sorrow commands their full attention. You may find yourself asking questions like the weary psalmist: *Is God angry with me? Where is God? Why did God let this happen?* Wayside soil doesn't breathe. Faith can be lost there. Even then it may be *solely* interpreted as a spiritual attack against their faith. Does the Enemy come to steal, kill, and destroy? Absolutely. Do we war with that Enemy? Absolutely. But your heart is *not* your enemy. Sadness is a signal that something valuable feels far away or has been lost. Sadness says you are disconnected, and you *need* connection. Attend to the need. Disconnection is a ground zero threat to relationships.

Anger: The Stony Soil

Another area of the field was stony. Here Eden's abundant crops once grew, but the meaningful productivity that purpose provides gave way to a frustrating failure to thrive. The fall from hope landed us in a rocky place.

Jesus described the stony heart as *offended* (Matt. 13:21). That equates to being *displeased*, *indignant*, *annoyed*, or *disapproving*. All those words describe forms of *anger* along with many more, including *rage*, *hatred*, *disgust*, and *irritability*. Anger is an emotion characterized by tension and hostility that urges us to act when we feel threatened. That action might just be a way of expressing our anger or it may be squarely directed *at* who or what made us angry.[2]

The desert sands.

If you have ever been to the desert (or the beach), you know that sand is just a bunch of tiny *stones*. It's literally stony ground. How does that help us understand anger? Sand has one thing in common with good ground: sand breathes. Remember that just as soil needs good airflow, we need faith to flow through our hearts. Air easily moves through sand particles. Anger and faith can be in the same place at the same time. The problem is that tiny rocks can't hold water or nutrients. Losing water means losing hope and love. To make matters worse, when the sun rides high, those little stones get hot. *Fast.* No matter who you are, there is a situation that—at its most intense point—can leave your anger hot, your hope drained, and your love lost.

In the parable, there is a little good dirt among the stones; that fertile soil had joy in the water. The seed finds it and quickly grows, but the roots are too shallow and dry to survive the sun's intense heat. The plant dies as quickly as it had grown. We find stony ground and this doomed plant personified in the life of the prophet Jonah. Jonah's story is brief, one act with four scenes.

1. God tells Jonah to go deliver a warning to the people in a city called Nineveh. Jonah doesn't do it. Instead, he hops on a boat going in the opposite direction, so God decides to arrest his attention by causing a storm that gets Jonah tossed overboard and swallowed by a "great fish" (1:17).
2. Jonah finds fish guts to be a highly undesirable environment. After three days inside the fish, Jonah signs on to God's plans. The fish spits him out onto the seashore. God repeats the original instructions and Jonah follows them to the letter.
3. Jonah tells the people in Nineveh that God is going to destroy

them because they were involved in some pretty nasty stuff. The people in Nineveh change their ways, and God showers them with mercy instead of wiping them out.

4. This makes Jonah very angry with God. He goes and sits down outside of the city to watch and see if maybe God will still destroy them. That doesn't happen. Instead, God shows mercy to Jonah by sending a plant to provide shade for him while he sits there, outside, fuming. The large, leafy plant quickly grows, but its roots are shallow. The next day, a worm chews into the plant's dry roots. The plant dies as quickly as it had grown. Jonah remains there, sweating on the outside and burning so hot with anger on the inside that he tells God that he would rather be dead. Jonah's angry heart was stony ground from the start.

Goal interrupted.

Anger does not always end badly and sometimes we do well to be angry, but the direct plant-link between Jonah's life and stony ground warns us about a specific type of anger that's been undermining the garden within since the fall: frustration.

When something blocks us from getting what we want or achieving what we set out to do, we call that *goal frustration*.[3] Frustration is a form of anger that blends annoyance and disappointment.[4] The disappointment is important to recognize because it explains why frustration skyrockets when hope evaporates. Anger increases persistence *when there is hope* that the goal can still be achieved, despite tribulation and persecution, but high anger plus low hope eventually equals "It's not worth it." We walk away.

When the goal is purpose-related, this frustration is even more dangerous because purpose is relational. It is the role we are gifted to play in the communities we are a part of. Be it your church, your workplace, or your neighborhood, if you feel your efforts are being thwarted by people in the community, frustration can undermine life in the purpose zone *and* the relationship zone. In that scenario, high anger plus low hope equals "I don't forgive you." That makes it pretty hard to serve.

Jonah didn't have a problem with being a prophet, he just didn't want to serve Nineveh, so he was willing to stop living on purpose when God told him to go to *that* community. Jonah didn't believe he was connected to them. Given Nineveh's history of violence and oppressing neighbors, he likely felt they deserved destruction rather than the love he knew God would offer. Jonah saw the Ninevites as "them," not "us." After three nights of fishy distress, Jonah did have a change in direction, but only a shallow change of heart. When God didn't destroy Nineveh, Jonah's hope quickly evaporated. Anger blinded him to their shared membership in the community of "*we* who need mercy," a community that includes us *all*. Goal frustration led Jonah to abandon his purpose. He decided he would rather die than continue to use his gift as a prophet.

Scripture reveals multiple examples of goal frustration disrupting purpose: Cain's anger led to the tragedies of murder and exile (Gen. 4:1–16). Moses' frustration with the people of Israel led him to respond poorly at a pivotal moment, leading to God barring him from the promised land (Num. 20:8–12). And Samson's temper famously led him into a series of self-destructive episodes (Judg. 13–16). Goal frustration is a ground zero threat to living on purpose.

Fear: The Thorny Soil

The barren wayside where disconnection saddens us and the stony ground that frustrates purpose reveal what was lost to sin, but in the legacy zone, something new appeared. Thorns started growing in the garden of Eden after the fall, and now our inner garden has weeds! Weeds are stubborn. They are also indicators. Remember how we learned about good ground based on what was growing there? According to the *Old Farmer's Almanac*, weeds have a story too.

When weeds arrive, it's often an index of what is wrong with the soil . . . They are a symptom . . . If we learn to read the weeds as clues to our soil's condition, we can help the soil recover.[5]

In the parable of the sower Jesus names our weeds. He says the thorns are the "anxiety of this age," "the deceitfulness of riches," and the "pleasures of this life" (Matt. 13:22 LSV; Luke 8:14).

How many times have you tried to stop your anxious thoughts from listing every possible outcome of a situation that may never occur? Or been overly focused on money so that you have the power to control what happens to you? Or activated your *I-know-it's-bad-for-me-but-it-feels-so-good* thing to avoid the pain of the moment? What do those thorns indicate about the soil's condition? Fear is the common thread. It's what's wrong with the soil in the thorny zone.

Fear is the impact of a situation that threatens to be painful. The pain can be physical or emotional. It can be actual, imagined, imminent, potential, short-term, or persistent so long as the situation involves uncertainty or limited control.[6] Each weed that Jesus named is a thought or behavior that can be guided by the emotion of fear.

Sowing in silt.

Silt is a kind of soil that teaches us about fear.

Like sand, silt lets air flow; fear is open to possibilities.

Like clay, silt holds water; fear is absolutely full of hope. Expectation is still hope, even when we expect something bad.[7]

At the same time, fear seems to avoid the pitfalls of sadness and anger. Silt and clay both get muddy, but silt is slippery when wet. Slipping could mean falling, but at least you're moving. Isn't that better than being stuck at a "pity party"? Fear also seems smarter than anger. Compared to losing your temper, isn't it *wise* to stay aware of what could go wrong? Fear deceives us by disguising itself in good intentions.

We tend to believe that in some situations, fear really does help us. Like clay, silt can nourish growth; fear will keep trying to create a solution. But that "growth" is deceptive. Yes, the sower's seed took root among thorns and was even developing fruit, but the good work ended abruptly before the fruit matured. Why? Fear can't nourish the fruit of God's word-seed. Fear only supports weeds.

Like your heart and mine, all soil is vulnerable. Silt is very fertile at first—but water breaks it down and carries pieces of it away. That's called erosion, and compared to clay and sand, silt is the *most* vulnerable. And, like all of us, the longer that silt is *overwhelmed* the weaker it gets. The erosion steals nutrients too. There is one type of plant that starts growing when soil loses nutrients: weeds. One of the most common soil conditions indicated by weeds is a nutrient deficiency. But wait. It gets worse.

> Fear can't nourish the fruit of God's word-seed. Fear only supports weeds.

The most important nutrient that your backyard garden needs is called nitrogen. As weeds grow, they weaken the other plants by quickly leeching nitrogen from the soil. Nitrogen is to a garden what love is to our hearts. Just as we are nothing without love, plants cannot thrive in nitrogen-deficient soil.[8] Where love is deficient, fear rises. First John 4:18 says, "There is no fear in love," so just as darkness exists only as the absence of light, fear exists only as the absence of love.

To feel fear is to feel nervous, terrified, helpless, insecure, inadequate, endangered, or panicked. Have you ever noticed that in the presence of God's love and in our healthy relationships, we have the opposite experience? We feel peaceful and protected. Love feels like tenderness, compassion, and care. Love nourishes this belief: *I am safe.* Fear awakens the opposite: *I am not safe.*

But wait. It gets worse again. In the books of Matthew and Luke the word *apopnigó* is used to describe what those thorny weeds did to the fruit of God's Word. *Apopnigó* is translated as "choked" but it can also mean "to drown."[9] How can thornbushes drown fruit? The weeds that fear grows are notoriously strong. Thornbush roots destroy the silt's weak structure. A deluge of water then easily washes everything away.

Our fragile legacy.

Our legacy is heavily influenced by our talents. A poet heals a heart a century later by expressing what someone else couldn't find words for. A woman with administrative talents links her capacity to legacy by working at a nonprofit. A musician, like my coworker Casey, builds a home studio to publish music that invites people into God's presence for decades. The legacy zone is thick with silty soil. What you are naturally good at—the talent you were born with—bears fruit here. It is the most fertile part of us, but because silt is highly unstable, it's also the most fragile.

When we nurture our hearts with the unconditional love of God and the support of our loved ones, our hearts whisper, *I am safe.* The full potential of our talents is nourished. But since the fall, our fertility is daily challenged by our fragility. We experience opportunities as threats that drain nutrients from our heart-soil. A promotion. A larger stage. A new contract. Before we know it, our anxious thoughts—dressed as perfectionism and imposter syndrome—are choking the life out of our legacy. Instead of flourishing with joy, we spend our time overestimating threats, underestimating ourselves, and competing with others for what God already said was ours. The weeds of fear are an invasive species. They were never meant to live in the garden within. Fear is a ground zero threat to legacy.

The Noble Ruins

When the first man and woman chose the forbidden fruit over the safety of God's love, everything changed. Eden had a well-watered garden. Now the flow of our emotional lives can feel totally unregulated. Depending on how much clay, sand, or silt is in the garden, sometimes there's not enough water; other times it rushes in too fast or won't drain. The destruction of Eden is evident in our hearts, but even so, we are noble ruins.

Just as we can see the majesty of ancient architectural wonders despite decay and disrepair, we all reflect the Creator's intentional work. Christian psychologist Mark McMinn said it beautifully:

> If we sit long enough to listen and we open our eyes wide enough, we hear and see the story of sin and redemption—the story of noble ruins—echoing in every corner of creation.[10]

Echoing in creation. That's for sure!

We can't wrap up this chapter without talking about the fourth type of ground in the parable. The good ground. *Good* simply means fertile. That's important. This isn't a simplistic binary between good ground and bad ground. You are not a dichotomy, all or nothing. Some areas of your heart may be perfectly fertile for something, yet another area of your heart-soil may need to be healed. That's what cultivating the heart is about. None of us is perfect.

We've seen how three soil types help us understand the ground of our hearts, but modern soil science identifies four types of soil—just like Jesus' parable![11] The fourth soil type is called *loam*. Loam is good ground. It's fertile soil. Yet loam is not an entirely different type of soil. Loam is the properly balanced combination of clay, sand, and silt.[12] Sand keeps the air flowing. Silt keeps the water flowing. Clay holds the nutrients.[13] Three-in-one is fertile ground.

There I see the noble ruins. In Genesis 1:26 God said, "Let *us* make man." We were created in the likeness of our triune God. The fall broke us, but that likeness is so deeply embedded, we could only break into *three* pieces. Good ground is what happens when the three soil types—each insufficient on its own—come together. That balanced loam is fertile, full of nutrients, and easy to work, like the good ground of Eden. For me, this might be the most profound revelation that creation gives us for understanding this parable.

Some of our hearts are sandy. Others have a lot of clay or silt. We can't just suddenly change that today. Soil develops over a long period of time. Rock particles break down. Organic matter (things that have died) are absorbed. Microorganisms bring life to the soil and sustain nutrients and energy. It's a *process*, not a recipe. We are who we are. But there is good gospel news. It turns out that "a soil's fertility . . . is easier to change than the soil's physical properties."[14] How does that translate to our heart-work? We embrace the instructions the Creator gave to the first man and the first woman. We get intentional about dressing and keeping the garden within (Gen. 2:15). Each day we work toward fertile ground. Where do we start? From wherever we are. Just like Casey.

Take care of garden within

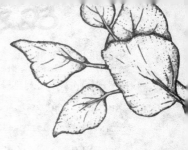

Chapter 5

HOW DOES YOUR GARDEN GROW?

> You crown the year with a bountiful harvest; even
> the hard pathways overflow with abundance.
>
> PSALM 65:11 NLT

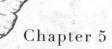

Tabitha Brown is one of my favorite influencers. She's a comedian, an actress, and the patron saint of vegan living. I am not a vegan, and I think that's true of many of the millions of people who follow her on social media. We just can't get enough of Tabitha's oh-so-infectious energy. She always brings inspiration no matter what she's communicating. At the same time, she has been open about the pain in her own life. It's the authenticity for me. The bright colors she wears, her Southern charm, and her unapologetic love for Jesus make her downright irresistible. An encounter with Tabitha's content feels like an encounter with pure joy. So when she launched her children's show, *Tab Time*, I watched that too (despite my age falling well outside the target demographic). The first episode became an instant favorite for me because Tab (and her buddy Avi the Avocado) taught us about how things grow.[1]

The episode begins in Ms. Tab's real-life garden. Then she and Avi whisk us off to a brightly animated fruit orchard where we meet an orange-tree seed named Marmalade. Marmalade tells us that all she needs to start growing is good ground and some water. Ms. Tab tucks Marmalade into

61

the soil and waters her well. Then we all pretend our arms are the arms of a clock; together, we speed up time by making big arm circles. A few seconds later Marmalade reappears, but now she is no longer a seed but a full-grown orange tree bearing her first fruit. Less than seven minutes into the episode, the preschool children for whom the show was created have already learned all they need to know to understand what you and I have been talking about for the last few chapters: how gardens grow.

The garden within may be a completely different way of thinking about how we were created and what it means to flourish, but when it comes to what you need to know to live this powerful life, you probably learned it in kindergarten or—at the latest—by the end of a middle school science class. The Creator made things very simple for us. No wonder Scripture encourages us to come to Jesus with the heart of a child (Mark 10:15). Things are so much easier when we do. And when it comes to letting the Creator change what we believe about how we feel, the timing couldn't be better.

It's Okay Not to Be Okay

When we catch a glimpse of Tabitha's real-life garden, it is too lush for words! It's full of bright colors and fruits and vegetables; this garden is *useful*. I don't know Tabitha personally, but I wouldn't be surprised if her garden looks exactly the way she wants her life to feel—a reflection of her goals for her garden within.

If you could design a garden that looked the way you want your life to feel, what would it look like? What would be growing there? Now ask yourself, *How is my inner garden looking?* Don't feel bad if the soil needs attention. Don't be surprised or upset if you notice that some areas are bare, some are growing well, and others are dying. You're not alone. In fact, a lot of people are not okay right now.

As I write these words, multiple global crises are affecting us all. It started in 2020 and it hasn't slowed down. I'm not just talking about the coronavirus. I'm talking about the mental health pandemic that it triggered. Covid-19 claimed a staggering number of lives in a very short period of time, leaving a trail of emotional devastation in its wake. With every death, an average of five loved ones are left grieving long-term.[2] That means that as of late 2022, more than thirty-three million people were grappling with the trauma attached to grieving someone who died not only unexpectedly but unimaginably, from a disease that seemed to come out of nowhere.[3]

There were other life-altering losses to grieve as well. So many of us missed attending not only funerals but weddings, baby showers, graduations, and milestone birthdays and anniversaries. These are the ceremonial moments that chart the timeline of our lives, shared memories that entwine us in relationship and in community.

On top of that, the way we understood and organized our lives fundamentally changed. People lost jobs. People lost homes. People lost businesses and dreams. People lost sobriety. People lost their sense of safety, and whether they have admitted it or not, some people lost their faith.

All that to say, a lot of people are not okay right now, and that likely includes you or someone you love very much. During 2020, global cases of major depressive disorder increased by 27.6 percent. That's an estimated 53.2 million more people than the year prior. Anxiety disorders increased by 25 percent. There was more anxiety to start with, so that increase amounted to around 76.2 million more people.[4] Of course, that's just counting the people we know about. So many others haven't sought help, so we don't have reliable confirmation. But like diabetes or heart disease, the diagnosis doesn't create reality; it just points it out. Maybe you haven't been formally diagnosed with depression, anxiety, or another mental health problem, but that doesn't mean what you are struggling with isn't real.

For the first time during my career, a significant number of mental health professionals have waiting lists. We can barely keep up with the demand. And from college kids to clergy, Christians are by no means exempt. At Christian colleges and universities, the number of students contacting campus counseling centers for issues like stress, depression, addictions, and suicidal thoughts also rose sharply.[5] The pastors striving to lead these young people as part of their congregations found themselves struggling too. In an October 2021 Barna study, pastors were asked to rate their well-being across six dimensions. Nearly a quarter of pastors surveyed identified as unhealthy overall, with emotional well-being the dimension most often rated as below average or poor.[6] Hear ye, hear ye! Knowing Jesus guarantees your salvation; it does not guarantee your emotional health.

Reflecting on the lack of emotional awareness in the body of Christ, author Peter Scazzero writes this in his incredibly important book *Emotionally Healthy Spirituality*:

> Christian spirituality, without an integration of emotional health, can be deadly—to yourself, your relationship with God, and the people around you. . . . Sad to say, that is the fruit of much of our discipleship in our churches.[7]

He goes on to say that "a failure to appreciate the biblical place of feelings within our larger Christian lives has done extensive damage, keeping free people in Christ in slavery."[8] As a therapist and as a minister, I see this over and over and over. Christians haven't had a scriptural model for understanding the critical role of the heart, so our response efforts have been unbalanced. But now you know that your emotional well-being influences every other dimension of your life, including your spirit.

Remember, the words of the kingdom are constantly being sown in the ground of your heart, so nourishing the fertility of that sacred seedbed is kingdom work. Living a powerful life requires you to embrace how your spirit, heart, mind, and behavior work together seamlessly. That means approaching your own heart as a garden rather than a war zone where you're constantly battling your emotions. Eden is our model for flourishing. The seeds of the garden of Eden were sown on good ground. I'm going to keep saying it—that ground is our hearts. Your heart is the soil of your life.

Your heart is the soil of your life.

Four Steps to Starting a Garden

As my understanding of the garden within has unfolded over the years (and continues to unfold), I constantly renew my commitment to keeping it simple. Everything I need to know about God's intentional work in planting the inner garden that I can't see is revealed in the gardens that I can see. When we ask how to begin the journey of intentionally cultivating the garden within, we don't have to look much farther than a garden near us to know how to get started. There are four steps to get a new garden growing.

1. Decide what you want to grow.
2. Prepare your location.
3. Set up a watering system.
4. Plant your seeds.

In this chapter we will follow these same steps to begin some intentional work in your own inner garden, and because I am ever a professor at heart, along the way we'll review what we've already learned. So pull out your journal, notebook, tablet, or notes app on your phone. Your garden needs a plan.

Step 1: Decide What You Want to Grow

Eden made this choice easy. In chapter 3 we learned that the original good ground was a blend of three life zones: the relationship zone, the purpose zone, and the legacy zone. Living a powerful life means cultivating a state of emotional well-being that catalyzes, sustains, and nourishes healthy relationships; productive, service-oriented purpose; and a love-fueled legacy that will outlast our time on earth.

If you are the type of person who likes to organize your journal entries with headings, you can title this one "Garden Goals." In chapter 3, you explored the good things already growing in each life zone. Give yourself a high five! Now let's think about what else you would like to grow. If you are still deciding, here are some prompts to get your wheels turning.

Relationship Zone Goals:

- What would I like to see newly flourishing in my relationship with myself?
- What would I like to see newly flourishing in my relationship with others?
- What would I like to see newly flourishing in my relationship with God?

Purpose Zone Goals:

- Which needs move my heart?
- Which gifts can I offer, big and small, to meet those needs?
- Which communities—which "we"—do I want to serve?

Legacy Zone Goals:

- What are my talents? What am I naturally good at?
- How can I use my talents to create things that will outlast my life on earth?

Step 2: Prepare Your Location

Jesus made it easy for us to know our garden's location. In the parable of the sower, Jesus told us directly that the ground is our hearts. In chapter 2 we learned that the seed-soil relationship is a Scripture-wide narrative, a love story that runs from Genesis to Revelation, and that it's the Creator's great hope for us to flourish as well-watered gardens spiritually, emotionally, mentally, and physically. But just because we know the location doesn't mean that our location-related work is done. Every good garden location needs some strategic preparation.

Remove the debris and the weeds.

The garden within is not a blank slate. You aren't starting from scratch. You have lived enough years and have enough life experience that your garden already exists. It may be a little overgrown, there are probably some weeds that need to be pulled, and there may even be trash lying around.

Intentionally cultivating your garden often requires you to remove some things. As Ecclesiastes 3:2 states, there is "a time to plant, and a time to pluck what is planted" (NKJV). Are there relationships, jobs, guilty pleasures, or distractions that need to be plucked? Identify them. Then elaborate. Be intentional about what steps are needed from you to successfully remove that person, place, or thing from your life.

Test your soil.

Preparing your heart for new growth includes checking on the soil. How do you feel about your garden goals? Maybe, like my coworker Casey, some of your goals are connected to tough emotions like shame or frustration. For the garden within, being good ground for what we intentionally choose to grow means cultivating emotional well-being. Cultivating emotional well-being begins with awareness.

Just as the easiest way to learn about the soil in any garden is to see how it feels, you can become more aware of your emotions by noticing how your body feels. Whether it's a stomach full of knots before a work presentation or full of butterflies before that third date, when emotions flow, your body feels it first. When we want to minimize or avoid our emotions, we often stifle the flow by ignoring our bodies. When we deliberately pay attention to our internal bodily sensations, we call that *body awareness*.[9] Body awareness is a garden tool we can use to test the soil. Let's try using it right now by deliberately paying attention to internal body sensations.

I hope you are excited to use this garden tool, but if not, I get it. Feeling *all* your feelings on purpose may sound scary. You might worry that any flow will quickly become a flood. I want you to know that any step is a step. Go at a pace that works for you. We're going to use *body awareness* to connect to our emotional pain and then lean into joy. Read all the instructions before you begin.*

1. Take a moment to recall a situation that you found moderately disturbing. On a scale of 0 (not painful) to 10 (extremely painful), begin with an experience that you would rate at 4 or 5. Think about the situation you chose. Close your eyes and notice any sensations you feel inside your body as you reflect on that memory. Make a note of what you notice in your body.
2. Now let's focus on joy. Take a moment to recall a situation that you really enjoyed or imagine a pleasurable experience that you hope to have. Close your eyes and spend time seeing yourself in the moment you chose. Holding that image in your mind, notice any sensations you feel inside your body. Make a note of what you notice in your body.

You just used your new garden tool! Keep practicing with different situations. Continue to notice what your body is doing and, as you feel ready, try sitting with those uncomfortable sensations a little bit longer each time. It gets less scary. This is one way of increasing our capacity to feel *all* our feelings—and that moves you closer to living your most powerful life.

Once you get the hang of using this tool, nurture the heart-spirit relationship by inviting the Creator's presence. You don't have to say anything. Just allow the Spirit to be there *with* you, especially when you

---

* If any painful feelings that you experienced during this activity go away by the time you complete the joy portion of the exercise, that indicates that you will likely be able to use techniques presented in the remaining activities in the book. In most cases, taking a few deep breaths and, if necessary, recalling an enjoyable experience will help to calm you sufficiently. However, if painful feelings do not easily resolve or you are currently in therapy for trauma recovery or a complex disorder (or suspect you would benefit from therapy for those reasons), other activities should be completed under the guidance of a state-licensed mental health professional. The guidance in this book is for general information purposes only.

touch pain. Finally, keep practicing joy too. Don't rush past it! Whether recalling a situation you experienced or imagining your hopes, linger there. Joy is good for us. When there is joy, hope is flowing.

Step 3: Set Up a Watering System

When I first introduced you to my pea plant, I told you that, while I loved her with all my heart, I didn't grow up to have a green thumb. I was being honest. My son and daughter will attest that in all their childhood years there was never a single living plant in our home. Seriously. I never even tried it. One year, when my daughter came to visit me for Mother's Day, she gifted me a stunning, oversized coffee-table book filled with colorful drawings of every type of flower you can imagine. It was the perfect gift for a woman who is always considering her inner garden. But the broad smile on my face quickly dissolved into confusion when she then also handed me a live potted plant. Before I could look up and ask her why she would endanger this lovely plant by placing it in my care, she quickly pointed out that the pot itself had a special water reservoir. It need be filled only once every few months. The soil would absorb water from the reservoir as needed. *Every few months?* I thought. *This plant might actually survive!* A self-watering system made all the difference for that plant. To intentionally cultivate your inner garden, you need to set up a watering system too.

When it comes to germination, different seeds have different needs. Some need only to come into contact with the soil surface. Others need to be planted deeper within the earth. Seeds have different temperature needs as well. And while most germinate in darkness, a few need light. Differences aside, we've learned that to come to life, all seeds need two things for sure: air and moisture. That's why fertile soil breathes, and fertile soil is well-watered. For any word-seed to become a living belief in your heart, it will need faith and feelings. Faith and feelings flow through the open spaces in the soil of your heart. As long as those spaces are open, the air replenishes itself. I mean, think about it. Have you ever checked on a house plant and thought, *This plant looks like it needs air.*

I better put some air on the soil. Nope. Never. The condition of the soil determines whether the air can get where it needs to be.

But we *do* expect to water it. Soil *needs* water. Maintaining soil moisture is an intentional act. So is maintaining your emotional well-being. Setting up a watering system for your inner garden translates to self-care. That's something else that you probably didn't know that you already knew. *Self-care is soil care.*

Consider your faith-related self-care practices, like prayer, reading Scripture, listening to worship music, or attending a church service. You know you need to breathe and that those practices sustain your faith. But consider how much those spiritual self-care practices impact the way you feel *emotionally*.

> Setting up a watering system for your inner garden translates to self-care.

Then there are other types of self-care activities, like spending time alone, making time for lunch with a friend, journaling, using your creative gifts, practicing gratitude, or playing with your pet. All those experiences help you to feel better.

Inconsistent, random acts of self-care aren't shown to help us much beyond that moment, just like a splash of water on dry soil won't save a plant's life. But research shows that self-care routines benefit us by increasing happiness; reducing stress, depression, and anxiety; and strengthening our relationships.[10] Those are emotional benefits. See? You already sensed that you are a garden. You already knew that you need a watering system. You already knew that self-care is soil care. Lean into that. Here are some questions and ideas to get you started.

- How do you regularly replenish yourself emotionally?
- How do you water your need for connection? For safety? For productivity? For creativity?
- What new activities would you like to incorporate into your watering system?

Step 4: Plant Your Seeds

A garden officially begins when a seed is sown and awakened. Those word-seeds can transform our lives for better or for worse. The apostle Peter told us that it is through the incorruptible seed of God's Word that we are born again (1 Peter 1:23). That's transformation for the better! Humanity was created in the image of God, so our words can also influence spiritual well-being. That's why Ephesians 4:29 says, "Let no corrupt communication proceed out of your mouth, but that which is good to the use of edifying, that it may minister grace unto the hearers." Proverbs 18:21 reminds us that our tongues can produce both life and death.

Bad word-seeds can do incredible spiritual damage. As a therapist, I've heard so many painful stories: A single woman whose mother told her that God will never give her a husband because she didn't remain a virgin. A pastor telling a woman that since her husband repented for molesting her young son, she had no grounds for divorce because God requires forgiveness. But the words don't have to be tied to religion to damage spiritual well-being. When a father tells his adult daughter that she was a mistake, or a teacher tells a student they will never amount to anything, the truth of our creation in God's image is challenged. Those wounds are spiritual too. Our spiritual well-being hinges on the quality of the word-seeds sown because they can determine what we believe is true about God and ourselves. Each seed is a potential blessing or a potential curse. I say *potential* because a seed is influenced by the soil it's planted in. The seed's power can only be unleashed by the soil.

What seeds do you have already? Here are some questions and prompts that can help you start that journey of assessing which seeds you already have, for better or worse.

- What do I believe about myself?
- What beliefs about myself am I struggling with?
- What do I believe about how God shows up in my life?
- What do I believe about how God sees me?
- What new beliefs would I like to plant instead?

Just for fun, here are a few more questions to help you articulate the words you believe:

- In my life, love is _____.
- The world around me is _____.
- To me, family is _____.
- When I cry, that means I am _____.
- In my life, joy is _____.

Now consider what new seeds you hope will take root in your garden. What do you want to believe about God, yourself, and others? What emotions make it hard to believe those words? What reasons do you have to be hopeful that those seeds may one day bear new fruit in your life?

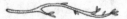

Transforming rough patches of soil takes time. As you begin to intentionally cultivate your garden, you don't need to rush. If you try to do all the things all at once, you may deplete the soil rather than restore it. Remember, this work is supposed to be a process. Your goal is to cultivate a sustainable, long-lasting garden. Cultivate the practice of slowing down.

Part 2

DEEPLY
ROOTED

In part 1 of this book, we emphasized the seed-soil relationship
to understand how our emotional health relates to our
spiritual health. We learned
that emotion is an active ingredient in our
spiritual lives. Now, for part 2 we will address
these pressing questions: What is the heart-
mind relationship? How does our emotional health
influence our mental health? In pursuit of a powerful life, how can heart-
work help us to renew our minds? The answers are in the garden.

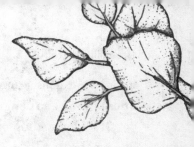
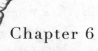

Chapter 6

WATER, WATER EVERYWHERE

One Sunday after church, a woman named Lena asked if she could walk with me to my car. She wanted to ask me for help. Actually, she hoped I could help her find a way to help her husband, John. She explained that during the previous six months, John's thinking had become increasingly negative. She was worried that John was giving up on trusting God. She had done her best to encourage him but to no avail. Lena knew I was both a minister and a therapist, so she was hoping I could recommend a Bible study they could do together, something focused on taking control of our thoughts and renewing our minds.

"What happened six months ago?" I asked.

Lena looked perplexed—like, hadn't she just told me? I clarified: "I mean, what else happened in your lives six months ago?"

It took Lena a few seconds to think about it. "Hmm . . . our son's longtime caregiver retired about eight months ago. She was so good! We finally found a replacement, but the search was a nightmare."

"What type of care does your son need?"

Lena let the whole story spill out. She explained that, as a child, John had survived cancer, but the treatment affected his fertility. They couldn't afford the expensive procedures that might have helped them conceive, but after praying and clinging to faith for a decade, they got pregnant.

"Finally holding our baby boy in our arms felt like standing in the sun for the first time in ten years," she said.

I noticed tears welling in Lena's eyes. I squeezed her hand as she continued to share. "Four years later everything went dark for us . . . again."

Their son, J. J., was diagnosed with a severe developmental disorder. Without another miracle, he would likely need care for his entire life. Lena and John were devastated, but they jumped right into action mode anyway. There was so much to learn and so much to do to give their son a chance at the best life possible. Their first caregiver was an incredible find, but even with her help John and Lena were often overwhelmed by financial worries and the physical exhaustion related to their beautiful son's care.

"I'm so sorry, Lena. Have you found ways to care for yourself in the midst of all of this?"

"Yes, I have made a point of doing that. I have close friends and we take good care of each other. They let me cry when I need to and help me stay positive."

Listening to Lena describe her friendships, I considered John's inner garden. I wondered what might be happening in his relationship zone.

"Does John spend time with friends as well?"

"He does have one good friend, but since J. J.'s diagnosis, John works a lot of overtime hours to cover everything, so he is usually too tired to hang out with anyone."

"Lena, here's my suggestion for you and John. Let's not focus on his negative thinking. It sounds like John is emotionally devastated. He hasn't had time or space to grieve J. J.'s diagnosis. There is a support group for parents of children with special needs that meets weekly at the library downtown. They also have a monthly gathering just for fathers. Try going to some meetings together. Pour your hearts out about everything in a room with people who intimately understand. Start there. The fathers-only events might be especially good for John."

Several months later, Lena greeted me with great news. Life

remained demanding, but John was sleeping better and laughing more. Lena and John had become very active in the parent support group. The new friendships formed there were transformative for John.

Inseparable

I love the garden model for understanding well-being because a garden is an interdependent, living system. The relationship between the seed and the soil informs a plant's growth and the fruit it produces. It's all connected. However, when it comes to our lives, we have been taught to understand ourselves as a collection of separate parts. Defining ourselves in this way isn't very helpful. We know that we have a spirit, a heart, a mind, and a body, but when it comes to taking care of ourselves, that knowledge is meaningless if we don't know how each part depends on the others. If you don't understand how your "parts" are interrelated and interdependent, you risk engaging in a futile internal war concerned only with how one part may be fighting another.

Many of us aren't used to thinking about systems, so let me give you an example of one that you might be more familiar with: an engine. The engine in my bright-blue car has about two hundred individual parts, but parts alone do not make an engine. They must be assembled and connected in the right relationships to become a system. When that system is properly fueled and activated, something emerges that no individual part had on its own: power. You must understand yourself as a system to tap into and wield your own emergent power.

Engines and gardens are both systems, but each part of an engine can exist on its own. If I take out the spark plug and lay it on the table, it's still a spark plug. A garden is a much more sensitive system. If I pull a plant out of the ground and lay it on the table, the plant will die. It cannot exist outside of the system. In the same way, your thoughts don't exist separately from your feelings. Your heart is the soil of your life. The roots of your mind are anchored there.

Renewing Your Mind

The Bible uses fruit to describe what we are *doing*. In my work as a therapist, my first question for a new client is, "Why did you decide to come and see me?" I am usually handed a basket of "fruit" containing a collection of painful behaviors that they want to change. Time and time again I hear some version of "I am doing this, and I don't want to anymore." People really do want to stop getting into toxic relationships, sabotaging their own dreams, relapsing into an addiction, or yelling at their kids. If their fruit is poisoning the people that they love, the distress is even greater. If it also contradicts their religious beliefs, another layer of shame may be added: "Why do I keep failing God like this?"

My second question is, "What have you already tried?" By the time most people ask for help, they have exhausted every strategy they could think of and are quickly losing hope. They have been thinking and doing and thinking again and doing and trying again to think differently but still producing the same doing. It's exhausting! Have you ever been there? Change can be really, really hard.

The first question my clients often have for me is some version of "How do I finally change?" If they grew up in church, they most likely learned that change comes through mind renewal because Romans 12:2 says, "Do not be conformed to this world, but be transformed by the renewing of your mind" (NKJV). So the question becomes "How do I renew my mind?" The answer they most likely learned is in 2 Corinthians 10:4–5, which says,

> For the weapons of our warfare are not carnal but mighty in God for pulling down strongholds, casting down arguments and every high thing that exalts itself against the knowledge of God, bringing every thought into captivity to the obedience of Christ. (NKJV)

And that's where things get sticky.

Prayer and reading Scripture are essential spiritual tools. Praise, worship, and fasting also empower us. Our spiritual practices are a super-natural arsenal, and with them we can accomplish what we could never do on our own. However, taking rogue thoughts captive can feel like the antithesis of supernatural work, and by the time many Christians show up in pastoral care or professional counseling, they are devastated that none of it seems to be working because they haven't changed or the change never seems to be "once and for all." Whether trying to *stop* doing something or *start* doing, they are usually focused on failing to renew their minds.

Things can get even harder when we try to change the way we *feel*. One of the lies we have been taught about emotion is that thoughts create feelings. That lie fuels the war against emotion and tells us that if we can use our thoughts to create feelings, we can use our thoughts to overthrow feelings. Neither is true, but based on that, so many sincere people of faith are living under condemnation for feeling anxious or depressed. The world we live in too often equates emotion with weakness. My clients who are Christians arrive carrying that stigma *plus* the belief that their emotional state is also a spiritual failure because they haven't been able to fully renew their minds.

When Lena spoke with me in the parking lot that Sunday, that was her fear for John—that he wasn't doing mind-renewing work. To her that meant putting negative thoughts out of his head and replacing them with positive thoughts that align with God's Word. Lena didn't yet understand the true nature of the relationship between our hearts and our minds.

The Heart-Mind Relationship

The relationship between your heart and your mind is the same as the relationship between soil and a plant. Just as the soil is there *before* the plant, feeling comes *before* thinking. Hearing that may be jarring; I understand. How often have you heard it said that your thoughts create your feelings? How many times have you tried to find peace by changing your thinking, only to have that fear or grief or anger fade temporarily

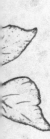

Just as the soil is there *before* the plant, feeling comes before thinking.

and then return stronger than ever? So many have reached the point of despair, wondering why they can't think their way out of feeling. The explanation is simple. We weren't created that way.

We hear this divine ordering echo across Scripture. In the original text of verses where both heart and mind are mentioned, we consistently find that the word translated as *heart* comes first; for better or worse, a matching mental state follows. Here are a few examples.

> But when his *heart* was lifted up, *and* his *mind* hardened in pride, he was deposed from his kingly throne, and they took his glory from him. (Dan. 5:20, emphasis added)

> And I will raise me up a faithful priest, that shall do according to that which is in mine *heart* and in my *mind*: and I will build him a sure house; and he shall walk before mine anointed for ever. (1 Sam. 2:35, emphasis added)

> And thou, Solomon my son, know thou the God of thy father, and serve him with a perfect *heart and* with a willing *mind*: for the LORD searcheth all *hearts, and* understandeth all the imaginations of the *thoughts*: if thou seek him, he will be found of thee; but if thou forsake him, he will cast thee off for ever. (1 Chron. 28:9, emphasis added)

> Jesus said unto him, Thou shalt love the Lord thy God with all thy *heart, and* with all thy soul, and with all thy *mind*. (Matt. 22:37, emphasis added)

In part 1 of this book, we explored scriptures where the heart's state influenced the *spirit*. We learned that our heart is the soil where spiritual seeds are planted. In these verses, we see a heart that is lifted up, open, willing, or loving that precedes a *mind* that is congruent. Your heart anchors the roots of your mind. Plants are stabilized by their soil. What's going on in the ground affects a plant's productivity, disease resistance, and stress tolerance.[1] That's exactly what your heart does for your mind.

What Can We Learn from Trees?

Do you remember when I mentioned that some neurons look like bushes or trees? The neuron in this picture is a perfect example. Look at the intimate craftmanship. It is truly beautiful. Named for the scientist who discovered them, these *Purkinje neurons* live in an area in the back of your brain called the *cerebellum*. The Creator planted a Purkinje neuron forest there. Why did the Creator shape neurons to look like trees? What lesson plan was He constructing? What do trees teach us about thinking?

A Purkinje Neuron

Thinking Begins with Believing

A tree grows from a seed. We know that seeds are words that, when awakened by fertile heart-soil, become beliefs. We already defined a belief as "acceptance of the truth, reality, or validity of something . . . particularly in the absence of substantiation."[2] All words are seeds, and the ones we accept as truth are part of our belief system. Our belief system determines our spiritual well-being.

Thinking Is Asking Questions

We can't see it with our naked eye, but the roots, trunk, branches, and leaves—which we collectively refer to as the tree itself—are always in motion. Like all plants, trees are always busy. Growing, making seeds, and creating fruit is hard work. Plants need energy for all of that, so they draw water and nutrients from the soil and then get light and air from the world around them to make their own food. That process is called *photosynthesis* and it goes on all day every day. If light is shining, plants are making food. We have a perpetual internal process too. Our process is called *thought*. Thought is "the process of thinking."[3]

How do I define thinking? As a Q&A session in your head.

Thinking is like photosynthesis, but instead of making food, we make the *answers* our minds are hungry for. You may have never noticed, but thinking is just *a series of questions* we ask ourselves from the moment we wake up until we are asleep again. If we are awake, we are probably making answers.

- **Daydreaming** is a form of thinking: What would it be like to live by the ocean? I'm sure John and Lena had a thought like this: What will it be like when we have a child of our own?
- **Imagining** is a form of thinking: What will happen if I say yes to this job offer? What will happen if I don't?
- **Problem-solving** is a form of thinking: Can I afford to replace that flat tire right now? If not, can another team mom drive my son to basketball practice until I get paid?

    Thinking is asking questions. You may produce the answers so quickly that you didn't notice the questions, but trust me, it was there. Some questions have been asked and answered so many times we don't ask anymore. Like, when was the last time you woke up and asked yourself, *Will I brush my teeth today?* Asked and answered countless times. We call that a habit. Sometimes the questions are so simple you barely notice them. *What do I feel like eating? What should I wear today? Which route should I take to get to work on time?* That's fast food. Those kinds of answers are easy to make. Others are much harder.

- **Meaning-making** is a form of thinking. An important form. Meaning-making refers to how we explain or make sense of things that happen.[4] When hard things happen, meaning-making questions proliferate. They often begin with "why."
  - Why can't I beat this addiction?
  - Why did God let this happen?
  - Why doesn't my partner love me anymore?
  - Why is my child suffering like this?

When we ask why, what we most often want to know is, "What does this *mean*[5]?" [5]We are asking how the relationships, places, and events in our lives are connected.[5] When something happens that violates every expectation—every hope—these questions can be insatiable; there may be no answer good enough to satisfy our mind's hunger. John's thoughts were filled with unanswered meaning-making questions about his son J. J.'s diagnosis.

Thinking Becomes Doing

A tree produces fruit. Fruit is *behavior*. A behavior is an activity "in response to external or internal stimuli."[6] Some behaviors are visible. If you jump up and down in front of me, I will see that behavior. Other behaviors are private events known only to you. Some, but not all, mental activities fall in that covert category.[7]

The way that fruit develops shows us why some changes are so hard. Fruit is a result. It is the outcome of a long process.[8] An almond tree can take five to twelve years to produce fruit for the first time. However, once a tree delivers its first harvest, it will produce the same fruit again and again if conditions remain the same. Our *doing* is the same way. That's why we get so frustrated trying to change a stubborn behavior by focusing on just the behavior itself. Fruit is the *end* of a process and, in dropping new seeds on the soil, that process becomes a cycle.

Free Flow

In chapter 2 we learned that water teaches us about the role that emotion plays in our inner garden. Plants wilt when they don't have enough water inside of them. That's because up to 95 percent of a plant's tissue is water![9] Just as water supports a plant's structure, our feelings shape our thoughts. Water is also essential to photosynthesis. In the same way, our emotions fuel our thinking process. When Lena shared her concern about John's thinking having become increasingly negative, I was immediately curious about his heart. Why? John's thoughts were wilting. He was losing hope. Without hope, we cannot experience joy.

When we are experiencing joy, our minds expand. Joy makes us more open to new information, and our problem-solving questions and answers become more creative. Have you ever been in a situation where the same thing went wrong again and again until you finally got so frustrated that you took over and solved the problem in two minutes? If so, you know that anger increases creative problem-solving too. However, research shows that while anger helps us solve problems faster, joy helps us solve them more accurately.[10]

Fear can make us more creative too. Most people don't like to say that they are afraid, so for the moment, let's use gentler language: *prevention-focused* (i.e., anxious or worried about something we don't want to happen). A study published in the *Journal of Personality and Social Psychology* found that prevention-focused states produce as many creative ideas as joy and anger, but joy and anger leave us inspired to move on to solving the next problem; we stay engaged. When fear—or rather, prevention-focus—finishes solving its problem, we disengage.[11] We don't want to think anymore! Fear eventually kills the plants.

Like fear, sadness is a painful emotion, but it influences the thinking process in a different way. Fear inspires a problem-solving Q&A focused on low-risk options even though low risk also means low reward. A Columbia Business School study found that sad individuals were far more likely than anxious individuals to seek high-reward outcomes.[12]

Whether it's sadness, fear, anger, or joy, what's in the water flows into the fruit. In fact, "water is the most abundant component of most fleshy fruits, and it is essential for fruit growth and quality formation."[13] Likewise, our behaviors reflect what's happening in the soil of our hearts. These twenty-first-century research studies offer great examples of lessons the Creator planted for us long ago.

In 2022, Dr. Leonard Mlodinow, a theoretical physicist, published *Emotional: How Feelings Shape Our Thinking*. In it, he explains that scientists have long "believed that rational thought was the dominant influence on our behavior and that when emotions played a role they were likely to be counterproductive."[14] However, "twenty-first-century technology has provided scientists with the means to look beyond the superficial aspects of emotion, with the result that the traditional theory of emotion has also been proven wrong."[15] The result is that

> The new science of emotion has expanded our self-knowledge. We now know that emotion is profoundly integrated into the neural circuits of our brains, inseparable from our circuits for "rational" thought. We could live without the ability to reason, but we would be completely dysfunctional if we couldn't feel. Emotion is a part of the mental machinery we share with all higher animals, but even more than rationality its role in our behavior is what sets us apart from them.[16]

Read that again. Many might assume that our minds separate us from other animals, but it turns out it's our hearts.

It's rare that the scientific community recognizes that a broad error has been made. The cutting-edge changes in emotion science that Dr. Mlodinow references began around 2010. These advances have confirmed that emotions are not the result of our thinking. Emotions *precede* other mental processes by subconsciously directing our attention and focus.[17] Science is catching up with the ancient wisdom of Scripture in recognizing that in the garden of our lives, our heart is indeed the soil where it all begins.

Even though it's been proven wrong, it may be decades before the newest scientific understanding of emotion changes the way the world feels about emotion now, but you don't have to wait for the culture to shift. You can flip the switch right now by following the example Jesus already set and by applying garden principles to the relationship between your heart and your mind.

When Lena stopped me in the church parking lot that Sunday, she seemed a bit angry. And she was, because on Saturday, during their morning prayer time, John had said that he felt unsure about continuing with their daily prayer for their son J. J.'s healing. That, combined with John's increasingly negative thinking, completely frustrated her. She was in full problem-solving mode when she came looking for me. She had a solution—help John renew his mind—but her solution wasn't accurate. Lena wasn't looking at what was happening to John's heart. She was distracted by his thoughts.

We all tend to look at what's happening on the outside, but God is always looking at the heart (1 Sam. 16:7). We can shift our attention to the heart by being curious about how people are feeling. We can listen for it in their thinking. When it comes to the critical role your emotional life plays in your inner garden, just remember this: water, water everywhere.

Zone Defense: The Relationship Zone

I don't want it to seem like I'm being hard on Lena. She and John were both dealing with their son's health issues in the best way they could. I am sure that Lena did consider how John's broken heart related to the changes she saw. Her error was believing that his mind was the best place to stage an intervention when it was in fact his heart. John was filled with deep sorrow. Sadness says, "I need connection."

Lena had a long-standing group of friends who rallied to support her; those connections kept the grass in her relationship zone thick and green. John's grass cover, however, was sparse from the start. Now the soil of his heart was bare and vulnerable. Working extra hours meant John had even less time for the one friend he did have, less time for his small group at church, and less time with Lena. And in the depths of grief, we tend to isolate ourselves while wrestling with our thoughts. John was wrestling. A lot.

Why did this happen to my son?

Are these the wrong treatment options?

Was it a mistake to opt out of the clinical trial?

Will my son ever know I love him?

All the questions were nurtured by sadness. Those plants soon crowded John's heart and threatened the very roots of his faith. John began feeling disconnected from God too. More isolation.

Have I misunderstood what the Bible says about healing?

If I feel doubt, isn't it better not to pray for healing until my faith is stronger?

Is God punishing me for how I am feeling?

But John needed something more than he needed those answers. He needed connection. The kind of connection that heals. It all came down to the soil of John's heart, and the grass there wasn't looking too green. The best play was to aggressively defend the relationship zone.

I knew that at the support group John and Lena would meet parents who knew what they were going through. In their stories, John's painful feelings and thoughts were normalized; he stopped being so hard on himself. I hoped that connecting with other fathers raising a child with special needs would add essential new friends. It did. John became close with one guy in particular. They started taking their wives on double dates and talking more vulnerably as couples. John didn't have to wrestle with his questions alone. From that couple, John and Lena both learned how to bring their messy feelings to each other and into the presence of God. That made all the difference. John needed safe relationships to help him navigate his pain. The relationship seed planted in John's heart at that first support group meeting was *"We understand."* His heart was good ground for that one.

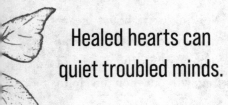

Healed hearts can quiet troubled minds.

We have been taught to believe that our mind is the ultimate refuge, but when it hurts this much, thinking rarely helps. These questions are watered by our pain. In those moments, we need healing more than we need answers. Healing for our grief. Our fear. Our fury. Healed hearts can quiet troubled minds.

Work the System

The Creator's brilliance is so clear in choosing to place a garden within each of us. A garden is a system we all understand. In every part of the globe, among every people group, against every cultural backdrop, across human history, people understand this system. We know the parts. We know the relationships. We know what can be produced. Seed, soil, plants, and fruit are all working together in a system. So is our spirit, heart, mind, and body. The war between the mind and the heart was not the Creator's design. Your mind is not meant to be a weapon against your feelings. Your heart nurtures your mind. Take good care of your heart and your mind will find rest. When the system is working in harmony, good things grow.

First we feel, then we think, then we do. Order mattered to God when He created the heavens and the earth, and as created beings, order also matters in the garden within. Understanding how God made you empowers you to live the life God intended you to live. When you realize the impact your emotional life has on every part of you, it becomes even clearer why the Bible says, "Guard your heart, for everything you do flows from it" (Prov. 4:23 NIV). You are always living from the heart, even when you don't realize it. Step one to renewing our minds is to know where we are emotionally and begin there. Renewing our minds actually begins with the heart: the soil where our thoughts are planted.

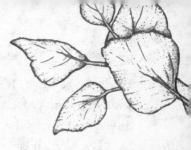

Chapter 7
DUST OF THE GROUND

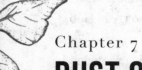

> And the Lord God formed man of the dust of
> the ground, and breathed into his nostrils the
> breath of life; and man became a living soul.
>
> Genesis 2:7

Ten minutes into our Tuesday morning session, my client's eyes filled with tears. He stopped talking for a moment to steady himself.

"Brian, what are you feeling right now?" I asked.

"Sadness," he replied. "Reflecting on that memory, seeing that image in my mind, I can feel the sadness of that moment."

I could have asked Brian to analyze why he felt sad instead of angry or even afraid, but that would have been an invitation for Brian to lose touch with that feeling of sadness and start thinking instead. He might have been grateful for the chance to escape his heart and return to the familiar, albeit tortured, terrain of his mind. But no such luck with me.

"Where in your body do you feel the sadness?" I asked.

"*Where in my body?*" Brian was incredulous. "What do you mean? All I ever feel in my body is pain."

Brian had been diagnosed with *dysautonomia*, a disorder of the autonomic nervous system. It left him suffering from extreme fatigue and chronic pain.[1]

It can be difficult to find an emotion—such as sadness—in the body amid the pain, especially when you aren't used to paying attention to it. So I stayed engaged with him in that moment.

"I can only imagine how hard it is to notice sadness when your body already hurts so much," I said. "Let's take a quiet moment to try to find it. Try closing your eyes and noticing what you feel in your arms, your chest, your stomach, your legs, or anywhere else. Now, holding that image in your mind again, where inside do you feel the sadness?"

After a moment, Brian said, "My head is getting heavier. My chest is getting tighter."

"There it is," I said gently. "You found it. Focus on those places."

Tears began streaming down Brian's face, and before long he audibly exhaled. I saw his shoulders drop. We let a bit of time pass in silence before I continued.

"Brian, what are you aware of in your body now?"

Brian's tone told me he was surprised. "The heaviness in my head and chest are gone. My chest feels light and open, and the pain I normally feel is so much better."

"Your pain level was a nine when the session started. Where is it now?" I asked.

"I'd say it's at about a three—which for me is incredible. I'm in intense pain so often, I would be happy to live my whole life at a three!"

We finished by exploring other times Brian may have noticed that his pain was more bearable. He recalled two emotionally fulfilling moments: a recent dinner with his wife and time spent holding his daughter on his lap.

Our emotions and our bodies are inseparable.

It was an important session. Experiencing the inextricable relationship between his emotions and his body changed Brian's feelings about his feelings. Our emotions and our bodies are inseparable. The soil teaches us about the heart, so we should not lose sight of the fact that the Creator made our bodies from that *same* soil.

Our emotions are embodied. We are embodied. There is no separation. It was true for Brian. It's true for me. It's true for you. It was true for Jesus.

Our Embodied Savior

It means so much to me that Jesus knows how I feel because He felt it, too, and now, having had the same experiences as me, He is praying for me every minute of every day (Heb. 7:25; Rom. 8:34). We can always pray with and for someone, no matter what is happening in their life. At the same time, there's something special about the way we pray for someone when we have experienced the same painful feelings they are having. That's how Jesus is praying for us. Jesus hasn't been in every situation we find ourselves in, but He has experienced every emotion (Heb. 4:15) because, as Philippians 2:7 says, Jesus "was made in the likeness of men." How? He put on a body.

It may have already been obvious to you that having a human body allowed Jesus to experience the same pain that we do when our flesh— our bodily tissue—is damaged. Every square centimeter of your skin has approximately two hundred pain receptors.[2] Jesus' skin did too. When He was slapped, whipped, and beaten beyond recognition, those pain receptors sent waves of fire through His body. As horrific as that was, tissue damage was not the only source of pain Jesus experienced. He also suffered emotionally. Jesus knows what emotional pain feels like for the same reason He knows what physical pain feels like. He knows because He had a body just like ours.

Sometimes emotional pain is a response to physical pain. It's easy to understand that someone like my client Brian, whose body constantly hurts, can become sad or irritable as a result. The fear that many people feel before having surgery is another example. That anxiety is often considered worse than the surgery itself.[3] Sadness, anger, and fear can all be responses to physical pain, but more often they are our response to the *social pain* of being rejected, abandoned, or devalued.[4] And "hurt" feelings do hurt. In 2010 a team of researchers representing six different universities tested the effects of pain medication to prove that social and physical pain rely on an overlapping set of neurobiological substrates.

> Daily doses of acetaminophen, a painkiller used to reduce physical pain, diminished daily psychological hurt feelings. Acetaminophen, compared with placebo, also decreased neural activity in response to social rejection in brain regions previously shown to be associated with experiencing social pain and the affective component of physical pain.[5]

An over-the-counter pain medication used regularly for headaches reduced the very real pain of rejection. *Emotion is a bodily experience.*

The Garden of Gethsemane

Jesus' crucifixion involved intense physical *and* social pain, so His bodily suffering began *before* a Roman soldier's whip ever landed on His back. It began in the garden of Gethsemane. Mark's gospel sets the scene: "They came to a place which was named Gethsemane: and he saith to his disciples, Sit ye here, while I shall pray" (14:32). Then Jesus took his inner circle, Peter, James, and John, deeper into the garden. Relationships mattered to Jesus. He didn't want to experience the social pain of being alone.

The Bible says that He "began to be sore amazed, and to be very heavy; and saith unto them, My soul is exceeding sorrowful unto death" (vv. 33–34). "Heavy"—*ademoneo*. That is the strongest of the three New Testament Greek words for depression.[6] Jesus felt *very* ademoneo and vulnerably shared His feelings with His friends. He told Peter, James, and John that His sorrow was so deep it felt like He was dying.[7]

That night in that garden Jesus experienced another feeling we are all familiar with: fear. Yes. I said it. The phrase "sore amazed" could literally be translated as *struck with terror.*[8] Why else would Jesus beg not to be crucified? Why didn't He just stroll over to Gethsemane and relax with the disciples until Judas arrived? Jesus wanted to escape such a gruesome, painful ending to His earthly life. He prayed, "Abba, Father, all things are possible unto thee; take away this cup from me: nevertheless not what I will, but what thou wilt" (Mark 14:36). My friends, this was not a reserved, contemplative prayer. Jesus prayed with "strong crying and tears unto him that was able to save him from death, and was heard in that he feared" (Heb. 5:7). Let me repeat two words: "Strong crying." This wasn't silent weeping. Jesus cried loudly.

The word translated "feared" in Hebrews 5:7 can mean reverence for God as well as fear, anxiety, or dread.[9] I believe that it meant both. Jesus "feared" God when He submitted His will as the Word to the Creator who speaks. Jesus was also experiencing fear in the emotional sense. We know this for two reasons.

The first reason is because that fear—that anxiety, that dread— showed up in His body. When we look at Luke's telling of Jesus' experience in the garden, we see that he included something Mark omitted: "And being in an agony he prayed more earnestly: and his sweat was as it were great drops of blood falling down to the ground" (Luke 22:44).

Jesus' body was reacting so strongly that blood vessels in His forehead were bursting. Blood mixed with the sweat that was pouring off Him. That is how intense His emotional pain was. This reaction, which doctors now call hematohidrosis, is rare, but it does happen. It is most commonly caused by acute fear when facing death or torture. Modern reported cases have included men sentenced to death and a woman in fear of being raped.[10] Jesus' bodily experience was inextricable from His emotional experience. Our bodies are the same.

The second reason we know Jesus was experiencing the emotion of fear is because that Hebrews verse also says that Jesus' prayer was "heard." Throughout Scripture, a prayer is described as heard when God grants the request.[11] We know that Jesus' request to avoid crucifixion was not granted, so in what sense was His prayer heard? His *heart* was heard. When we are afraid, we need to feel safe. The Father ministered to Jesus' need.

Luke 22:43 says that an angel from heaven appeared to Him and strengthened Him in that moment of human weakness. Jesus kept praying, and sweating blood, and getting stronger. When He stood up, fear was gone and, well, you know the rest. Jesus waited for the soldiers to get up after they were knocked to the ground by the power of His words: "*I am he*" (John 18:6, emphasis added). This is one of the most powerful moments of Jesus' earthly life.

Our Embodied Emotions

Embodiment is central to what it means to be human. Jesus had to put on a body like ours to have an experience like ours, including our emotional experiences. For Jesus to be made in the "likeness of men" was to be embodied. The emotions that Jesus encountered in Gethsemane were not a product of "stinking thinking." Those emotions were bodily experiences. And Jesus' response exemplified the definition of emotional well-being. We saw His capacity—and willingness—to be aware of, acknowledge, and experience all His emotions.

Historically, Western psychology has ignored the role of the body in the human experience of emotions. The tradition has *psychologized* emotion, as if emotions are things we create in our heads. Through that lens, emotion is often seen as something that's not quite real. When painful emotion shows up in the body, the way that it did for Jesus when His emotional distress manifested as sweat and blood, Western psychology describes that as *somatization*. The root word *soma* is a Greek word for "body."[12] Early on I was taught that somatization was a bad thing, an indication of pathology. It's not.

My client Brian, who also follows Jesus, had absorbed the psychologized view of emotion, so he was skeptical (you should have seen his face) when I invited him to embody his emotion instead. Brian is also intellectually brilliant, so stepping outside of his mind felt risky. I was deeply moved to see him have that experience for the first time and to see him realize that relief from his pain might be possible when he includes his body in his overall understanding of how he was created.

Although Brian may have still had a long healing journey ahead, finding out that he could release pain from his body by embracing his emotions *as a presence in his body* gave him the glimpse of hope he needed after suffering for so long. We don't look for things where we don't expect to find them, right? But the bodily sensations caused by your emotions are there. Now that we know emotion is carried and felt in our bodies, not something made up in our heads, let's officially define it that way.

emotion [ih-moh-shuhn] noun
The impact a situation has on your body and your brain.[13]

That's it. Plain. Simple.

The Sweet-Potato-Rum-Smell Near-Death Experience

I have always been afraid to use drugs. My sister's addiction really scared me, so growing up I was never tempted to experiment. My parents also raised us not to drink at all. Then I went away to college. I can still remember that first drink; my body soaked it up like water on dry ground. Muscle tension I didn't even know existed suddenly dissolved. I didn't know it at the time, but my body was holding *a lot* of emotional pain from traumas I had already survived. Before I was ever aware of those feelings, I packed my pain away, assuming I wasn't "the emotional type." But guess what? We all are. Add the emotional baggage stuffed into every corner and crevice of my body to a genetic predisposition for addiction, and I was an alcoholic waiting to happen.[14] I spent freshman year developing a serious drinking habit very quickly. A few months in, I almost died of alcohol poisoning after ingesting an inordinate amount of rum. It's a miracle I survived.

Five years later I was enjoying Thanksgiving with a friend's family. By then, I hadn't had a drink in two years. Everything on the table looked delicious, but when the whipped sweet potatoes were passed to me, the smell made me both nauseous and anxious. I didn't eat any and two days later I realized why. Rum flavoring! The smell took my body back to that devastating college night. I re-experienced *the impact that situation had on my body and my brain.* Fear. That had been a really scary night. My body remembered.

"Bodily experiences such as the feeling of touch, pain, or inner signals of the body are deeply emotional."[15] If you have ever had an experience like mine, where a smell or a sound or a sight brought back an awful feeling, then you already know that your emotions are bodily experiences. Our bodies remember the pleasures of joy and comfort too. If a certain scent relaxes you because it immediately reminds you of your first apartment that you loved or your grandmother's cozy house, you already know that emotion is a bodily experience; you just didn't know you knew it. And you already know that you don't have to *think* to re-experience those feelings. It happens automatically. That's because emotions—the impact that a situation has on your body and brain—are mediated by your body's autonomic nervous system (ANS).

That word *autonomic* is exactly what it sounds like: *automatic.* This part of your nervous system doesn't depend on your mind. It is responsible for things like keeping your heart beating, digesting food, and breathing. These processes happen when you're awake. They happen when you're asleep. They happen when you're happy. They happen when you're sad. You don't get to use your mind to decide to make your heart stop beating. You can't use your mind to decide to hold your breath for an hour. Well, you can try, but it won't be long before your ANS overthrows your efforts.[16]

The ANS regulates the systems that keep you alive. It also strives to keep you alive by keeping you safe. Your ANS is constantly scanning your body and your environment to assess your safety.[17] The nausea and fear I re-experienced in response to the scent of rum—five years after that night of poor decision-making—was my autonomic nervous system trying to protect me from a threat. The original impact had been memorized, and my ANS had reason to believe I might be in danger before my mind knew what was happening. We call that *neuroception.*

The neurons in the ANS operate beneath our awareness. Sometimes we can bring conscious *perception* to neuroception (like when my mind

DUST OF THE GROUND

put together the sweet-potato-rum-smell near-death-experience link two days later), but long before perception comes into play (if it ever does), the autonomic nervous system is working underground trying to keep us safe from both physical and emotional pain.

Learning about your nervous system will help you better understand your inner garden. It will further equip you to end the war with your emotions and begin living your most powerful life. The autonomic nervous system has two divisions: the sympathetic nervous system and the parasympathetic nervous system. For now, let's focus on the sympathetic nervous system.

Fight or Flight

When we sense that we are in a threatening situation, we usually become angry or afraid. It could be a physically painful threat, like encountering a venomous snake while hiking in the woods or an earthquake shaking your house. Or the situation may be emotionally upsetting, like seeing someone bully a young child or waiting for your doctor to call with the results of a medical test.

Under threat, neuroception immediately sounds the alarm, and the *sympathetic* nervous system (SNS) initiates what is popularly called the fight-or-flight response. Anger most often invokes the fight response (even when we keep the anger inside ourselves). When we are scared, we try to escape the situation (flight) or fight until we are safe again. In both cases, SNS activation means you breathe faster, your heartbeat speeds up, and your digestive system gets upset. Those changes create the bodily sensations you associate with both fury and fear.[18]

Emotion begins in the body, not the mind.

We are embodied. Our emotions are embodied. There is no separation. It's true for me. It's true for you. It was true for Jesus. And it was true for the apostle Paul, who had some very distressing experiences with his own sympathetic nervous system.

Emotion begins in the body, not the mind.

No-Judgment Zone

The apostle Paul wrote fourteen of the twenty-seven books of the New Testament. He was an influential Christian leader and a man of integrity who obeyed the Law and faithfully kept the Ten Commandments. His inspired words are still changing lives today. But there was something *within* Paul that he struggled with.

Paul's letter to the church in Rome tells the story. He wrote,

> For I know that in me (that is, in my flesh,) dwelleth no good thing: for to will is present with me; but how to perform that which is good I find not. For the good that I would I do not: but the evil which I would not, that I do. Now if I do that I would not, it is no more I that do it, but sin that dwelleth in me. (Rom 7:18–20)

Long before neurobiologists fully understood the sympathetic nervous system, Paul knew what it felt like for his body to overthrow his mind. Continuing, he wrote,

> For I delight in the law of God after the inward man: but I see another law in my members, warring against the law of my mind, and bringing me into captivity to the law of sin which is in my members. (vv. 22–23)

In these passages, I'm not convinced that Paul's main focus was on *behaviors* that break the Law of God, because in Philippians 3:5, Paul said he had followed the Law perfectly. When he said his mind was taken captive, I believe Paul was emphasizing an *internal* struggle. An emotionally painful one.

That word "members" (v. 23) literally means *body parts*. In the New International Version, it says, "I see another law at work in *me*" (emphasis added), but it's important to recognize that Paul was struggling with his body, not his character. I believe Paul's struggle was less about something he didn't want to do and more about something he didn't want to *feel*.[*] Emotional experiences begin in the body. Painful emotional experiences begin in the sympathetic nervous system.

Paul went on to offer both a lament and a reassurance:

> O wretched man that I am! who shall deliver me from the body of this death? I thank God through Jesus Christ our Lord. So then with the mind I myself serve the law of God; but with the flesh the law of sin.

> There is therefore now no condemnation to them which are in Christ Jesus, who walk not after the flesh, but after the Spirit. For the law of the Spirit of life in Christ Jesus hath made me free from the law of sin and death. (Romans 7:24–8:2)

I want to be clear that this does not make your body the enemy. Our bodies carry the consequences of the fall. In Genesis 3, after the first man and the first woman ate the forbidden fruit, the garden's ground changed. Painful emotional experiences emerged as wayside, stony, and thorny ground. Our bodies were formed from the dust of that *same ground*, so after the fall our bodies were different too. But our bodies are also the temple of the Holy Spirit. The Holy Spirit—God Himself—still desires and chooses to dwell within us. There will still be pain and struggles but you don't have to feel shame or condemnation on days when, like Paul, your mind doesn't end up ruling the day.

---

* We will explore Paul's internal tensions more deeply in chapter 14.

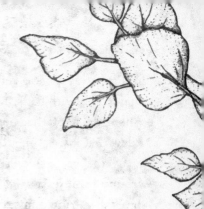

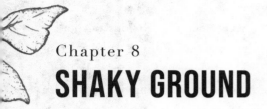

Chapter 8

SHAKY GROUND

> The LORD is near to the brokenhearted
> and saves the crushed in spirit.
>
> PSALM 34:18 ESV

Scott, a forty-five-year-old soldier, was relieved to be returning home to his wife and two children after the war in Afghanistan ended. But the hypervigilance that kept him alive during war—constantly assessing for potential threats around him—began to interfere with his relationships at home. He found himself needing to drink four to six beers at night just so he could fall asleep. His wife didn't like how much he was drinking, but it was the only time he was relaxed enough to engage in conversation. But when he exploded in anger after the noise of a nail gun his son was using in the garage startled him, Scott decided it was time to talk to a professional.

Jessica, a twenty-nine-year-old financial advisor, began noticing that she was experiencing emotional distress. She described having a happy marriage but over the course of two months noticed herself withdrawing from her husband without any explanation and found herself sleeping on the couch most nights out of the week. Her husband also pointed out that she had become extremely overprotective of their five-year-old daughter, and this was causing tension in their parenting decisions. When Jessica shared this with her sister, her sister reminded her that she had been five when her stepfather began abusing her. She broke down in tears and knew that it was time to go to therapy.

Scott was a soldier; his traumatic experience was obvious to those around him. Jessica believed she had left her trauma in the past years ago only to find it invading the new life she had worked so hard to build. Sometimes we're keenly aware of the traumas we've endured, and other times they lie beneath our conscious awareness.

I can't remember the first time I heard the word *trauma* in the context of emotional and mental health, but these days, it's hard to imagine that there is anyone who has *not* heard it. This widespread awareness is a good thing because trauma is an issue that has almost certainly touched your life or the life of someone you love. Trauma can affect anyone. No one is exempt.

The Substance Abuse and Mental Health Services Administration (SAMHSA) defines trauma as the "results from an event, series of events, or set of circumstances that is experienced by an individual as physically or emotionally harmful or threatening and that has lasting adverse effects on the individual's functioning and physical, social, emotional, or spiritual wellbeing."[1] That definition presents a three-dimensional view of trauma: the event, the harm, and the effects. In this chapter we will look at different sources of trauma, how they impact our lives, and what we can do to recover.

What *Happened* to You?

In 2022 the National Council for Mental Wellbeing reported that 223.4 million people living in the United States had experienced one or more traumatizing events.[2] That amounts to 70 percent of the country's population, which is on par with rates worldwide. Among 68,894 adults across six continents, the World Mental Health Survey Consortium found that more than 70 percent of them had experienced a traumatic event; 30 percent had experienced at least four.[3] Because of the widespread effects of trauma, many professionals and organizations that serve people—including schools, hospitals, churches, and behavioral health organizations—have adopted a trauma-informed approach to their work. The trauma-informed approach is guided by a single compassionate question: What *happened* to you?[4] Knowing what happened to someone can help us to understand why they may behave in certain ways or struggle with certain things.

Traumatic events occur all around us every day. They can be adverse childhood experiences such as physical, emotional, or sexual abuse; your parents' divorce; living with a sibling who has a mental illness; having a parent who struggled with substance abuse; or witnessing domestic violence. Traumatic events can include violent interpersonal relationships between spouses or romantic partners, and elder abuse.

Some traumatizing events affect many people at once.[5] Natural disasters like the 2004 Indian Ocean tsunami and human-caused disasters like the Russian invasion of Ukraine impact masses. An entire community can suffer from trauma after a local school shooting.[6] Some people are exposed to more traumatic events because they are part of a group whose work makes them vulnerable like firefighters or emergency room nurses.

Trauma can even impact the heritage of a culture through prejudice, disenfranchisement, and health inequities.[7] Some historically traumatic events can be so widespread, "they not only impact entire cultures, but they are so intense they influence generations beyond those who experienced them directly."[8] The enslavement and lynching of African Americans, the genocide in Rwanda, Japanese internment camps in America, and the Holocaust are all examples of historical trauma. When we explore widespread challenges faced by disenfranchised groups, a trauma-informed approach may ask, "What happened to *all* of you?"

What Happened to *You?*

The second dimension in our definition of trauma is effect. It is important to distinguish between the effects of the trauma and the traumatizing event. The effect is the wound the event leaves behind.

In chapter 7 we learned that be it the origination, manifestation, awareness, or experience of emotion, the autonomic nervous system (ANS) plays a critical role.[9] The sympathetic nervous system (SNS) automatically activates when our bodies are impacted by physical pain or the social pain of disconnection, threats, or the loss of control that traumatizing situations bring. Stress-related chemicals flood our body and brain. The problem is, the sympathetic nervous system doesn't have an "off" switch.

When the stressful or traumatic situation resolves, the SNS will keep running unless another ANS division intervenes to bring the body back into a state of calm. That intervening system is the parasympathetic nervous system (PNS). Together the sympathetic and parasympathetic subsystems ensure the body responds to meet different needs in a life-sustaining way.[10] When our nervous system is healthy, we are able to respond to threats and move through emotional pain because PNS activation enables emotional regulation. It restores equanimity and brings us into an emotional state of safety, peace, connection, and productivity. *Emotional regulation* is "the ability of an individual to modulate an emotion or set of emotions."[11] In garden language that means being intentional about the water flow. With water there are always questions of flow speed, depth, and temperature.

Trauma changes things. It's an earthquake that shakes our inner garden. And just as earthquakes have aftershocks, the effects of trauma can extend decades into the future as reduced stress tolerance, new triggers, and unwanted behaviors, leaving us struggling to live life on shaky ground.

Window of Tolerance

We all have what is called a "window of tolerance" for our capacity to handle stress. When we are regulated, we are within our window.

Stressful things like schedule changes, getting sick, or being late for an appointment may feel frustrating, but we are able to manage them without being overwhelmed. After experiencing a trauma, emotional regulation can become challenging because trauma changes our nervous system. The sympathetic nervous system becomes dominant, and our window of tolerance shrinks, sometimes quite dramatically. So those once manageable stressors start to fall outside of our ability to handle them.

Triggers

In her book *Why Am I Like This? How to Break Cycles, Heal from Trauma, and Restore Your Faith*, trauma therapist Kobe Campbell explains that "triggers are biological and relational reminders that something painful and confusing happened to us or around us in a way that affects our present experiences. They are evidence that our bodies store memories of the pain we've endured, even when those painful moments are long gone."[12] Those triggers can be obvious reminders such as a news report of an assault or suicide. Others are more nuanced, like a smell, a song, or an area of your home that reminds you of the traumatic event in some way. Your body and nervous system react as if you are re-experiencing that earthquake all over again. For Scott, it was the sound of the nail gun. For Jessica, it was the age of her daughter.

Unwanted Behavior

Trauma survivors may find themselves feeling trapped in a cycle of unwanted behaviors. Scott didn't want to need alcohol to fall asleep every night, and Jessica was tormented by the fears for her daughter that made her overprotective. Unwanted behaviors often arise from both conscious and unconscious efforts to regulate a wounded nervous system. That may look like withdrawing from social settings, feeling distrustful toward others, developing unhealthy sleeping or eating habits, succumbing to addictions, or throwing yourself into work as a form of avoidance.

Acknowledging the Pain

It can be difficult to acknowledge that we experienced a trauma. Acknowledging a wound from a past event can leave us feeling vulnerable and disempowered, but it simply means that we are human. If the trauma you suffered doesn't seem significant in comparison to someone else's, it becomes even harder to address, but traumatic events come in many shapes.

The child who had to "grow up too fast" and began shouldering responsibilities too early may become the adult who has a difficult time asking for help or truly trusting the available support around them. The kid who grew up with unrelenting standards of academic achievement often grows up to be a perfectionist, hypercritical of themselves and others. The child whose dad said one thing but did another may grow up believing they can't rely on anyone. Children who grew up believing their parents were not proud of them become adults who believe that they are unwanted or unlovable. These types of traumatic events leave wounds that we call *developmental trauma*. Rather than being characterized by a single event that *did* happen, developmental traumas are the result of what *didn't* happen for a child.

Even if you're still working to connect the dots in your own life between your childhood and your present, know that your experiences in childhood become the lens through which you see yourself, others, and God. Just because you weren't beaten, sexually violated, or verbally abused doesn't mean you haven't experienced trauma. I give you permission to embrace whatever *you* experienced.

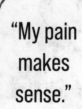

"My pain makes sense."

In order to recover and start the healing process, it is paramount to begin by simply calling it what it is. Consider this statement: "My pain makes sense." If that resonates with you, try reading that sentence out loud. Hear yourself say it. It's okay to acknowledge that during those childhood years something hurt you. You don't have to reject all the good things in your childhood or your adult life to also acknowledge that you may need to heal and that you are worthy of healing.

Healing Your Nervous System

At the biological level, healing the wounds of trauma is rooted in healing the autonomic nervous system. In a traumatized ANS, emotional dysregulation is characterized by a sympathetic nervous system that has been working overtime trying to keep you safe. The parasympathetic nervous system may need to be strengthened in order to reengage emotional regulation. Here are some ways to begin that healing process.

Create Safe Spaces

Your ANS is dedicated to keeping you safe. After a trauma hypervigilance is common, which means survivors may feel anxious on some level nearly all the time. Drawing boundaries to create safe spaces and spend time with safe people makes room for your body to begin adjusting to what safety feels like. Safety may be so new that it's uncomfortable but stick around—it will grow on you! You are allowed to remove toxic people and places from your life.

One of the best ways to do this is to be intentional about carving out time in your schedule to get some quiet and some calm in your environment. Where can you go to just *be*? No expectations. No agenda. Just peace and quiet. If you don't have a place, I encourage you to explore. It could be a park, a trail, a lake, your bedroom, your backyard, even your car. Find what works for you. And when you are ready, invite your safe people to join you.

Connect with Your Body

Trauma can be biologically overwhelming, causing us to lose touch with our own bodies. That means that we become less aware of how our body is feeling, so we lose touch with our own wants and needs. One way to reconnect is engaging in some form of physical movement. It doesn't have to be hard exercise. Some good options are walking, swimming, stretching, and dancing.

Build Community

Like John and Lena, you may find that being in community with others who intimately understand what you have experienced creates a special sense of safety where you may begin telling your story. The reclamation of voice is incredibly empowering. Support groups are a wonderful resource. You may be surprised to find how many different and specific groups are available. Trauma attempts to disconnect us from others and causes us to want to isolate. Simply being around others and engaging in relationship can begin to restabilize the shaken ground of your heart.

Work with a Trauma Therapist

There are many wonderful therapists waiting right now to hear from you. If you are a trauma survivor, I encourage you to search for a therapist who specializes in trauma work. There are many different approaches that a trauma therapist may use. Here are two approaches you may not have heard of. Both emphasize healing the autonomic nervous system.

Somatic Experiencing

The somatic experiencing (SE) approach to trauma recovery "works to release the [body's] stored energy [i.e., suppressed emotion] and turn off the threat alarm that causes dysregulation."[13] In the process, SE therapists gently guide and support clients as they increase their window of tolerance and more easily recognize the bodily sensations associated with their emotions. The key is to allow the client to process a difficult event from their past without retraumatizing them.

Eye Movement Desensitization and Reprocessing (EMDR)

EMDR therapy is an eight-phase treatment approach to trauma recovery that enables people to heal from the symptoms and emotional distress arising from disturbing life experiences. "After the clinician has determined which memory to target first, he asks the client to hold different aspects of that event or thought in mind and to use his eyes to track the therapist's hand as it moves back and forth across the client's field of vision. Internal associations arise and the clients begin to process the memory and disturbing feelings. In successful EMDR therapy, the meaning of painful events is transformed on an emotional level."[14] The parasympathetic nervous system is activated during this process. EMDR is not a form of hypnosis. When the process is complete, clients still remember the event; it just doesn't hurt anymore.

Bibliotherapy

There are also many wonderful books that have been written to support individuals on their trauma recovery journey, both as preparation for and alongside work with a licensed trauma therapist. Here are a few that I recommend.

- *Homecoming: Overcome Fear and Trauma to Reclaim Your Whole, Authentic Self*, by Dr. Thema Bryant, a clinical psychologist and elected president of the American Psychological Association in 2023, provides a road map for dealing with the fears and shame that keep us from living a free, authentic life.
- *Healing Trauma: A Pioneering Program for Restoring the Wisdom of the Body*, by therapist Peter A. Levine, normalizes traumatic symptoms and shows the steps needed to heal them.
- *Why Am I Like This?: How to Break Cycles, Heal from Trauma, and Restore Your Faith*, by seminary-trained, licensed trauma therapist Kobe Campbell, helps readers understand why it's so difficult to break the patterns of brokenness in our lives.

While not all of these books were written from a faith perspective, each offers valuable information. Embrace what blesses you and leave the rest behind.

A Message About Trauma and Faith

Many people struggle with the pain in this world and the idea of a good God existing in the midst of that. It is often said that everything happens for a reason. I believe that everything happens for a reason, but it's not always a good reason. Our Creator doesn't create chaos or cause trauma to happen to accomplish a grand purpose in our lives.

He doesn't need to do that. He can't do that because 1 John 1:5 says, "This then is the message which we have heard of him, and declare unto you, that God is light, and in him is no darkness at all." God does not have darkness to give us.

Trauma leaves us with many hard questions. Meaning-making questions about why you were targeted for the sex abuse, or why your parents got a divorce, or why your dad passed away, or why your friend died by suicide. In my faith tradition, I find my answer in Scripture. The Enemy entered the garden of Eden to cause suffering and destruction, and the garden wasn't his last appearance. First John 3:8 tells us that sin is in the world because of Satan, but for this purpose was the Son of God manifested: to *destroy* the work of the Enemy. Healing is a powerful way to destroy that work!

> I believe that everything happens for a reason, but it's not always a good reason.

You have been known to God from the womb, and you are still the divinely designed creation you have always been. Nothing can change that. Trauma may have shaped you, but it didn't make you. God made you and you are still exactly who God created you to be.

Though the abuse is in the past, where the effects remain present, where the ground continues to shake, and where the water may continue to rage inside of us, we can say, "Peace, be still." We can speak it in our spirits, live it in relationships, strengthen it in therapy, and nurture it in our bodies. The ground in us may have been shaken and we may be used to living in the aftermath of its quake, but our God is a rebuilder of ancient ruins and restorer of age-old foundations—even within you.

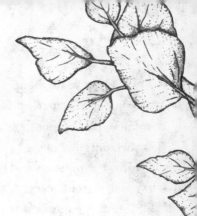

Chapter 9
WILDERNESS

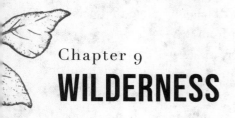

> I will plant in the wilderness the cedar and the acacia tree,
> The myrtle and the oil tree;
> I will set in the desert the cypress tree and the pine
> And the box tree together, that they may see and know,
> And consider and understand together,
> That the hand of the Lord has done this,
> And the Holy One of Israel has created it.
>
> ISAIAH 41:19–20 NKJV

From the age of five, my sister, Valerie, was experiencing hallucinations. A part of her body was already broken: her brain. And as she got older, schizophrenia and addiction held her captive for devastating stretches of time. While my family now understands Valerie's suffering, mental health and illness wasn't a conversation that was happening in our community at the time.

The need to acknowledge and understand mental illness is not limited to religious circles or any other segment of society. It is an issue everywhere. Even though the causes are often organic, as with the chemical imbalance in Valerie's brain, people often view mental distress and physical distress differently. For example, when a person has a stroke, they may lose their ability to speak. They haven't decided that they don't want to talk anymore. There's nothing volitional about it. We don't blame or judge that person for having had a stroke. Dementia is similar. We know that dementia is eating away at a loved one's brain; we know that their mind is being taken captive. We don't blame or judge that person for the symptoms and behaviors that result from it.

In recent years our culture has been increasingly willing to pay attention to mental health issues. Slowly but surely, we're doing better. But there is still a very present prejudice in our society against people who suffer from mental illness. Attitudes and assumptions of shame, blame, incompetency, punishment, and criminality toward people with mental illness are common. Over one-third of Americans are likely to report avoiding a person with mental illness.[1] Children with mental illness (for example, depression or ADHD) are more likely to be viewed as lazy compared to children with other health conditions.

Mental Illness vs. Physical Illness

Categorizing illness as strictly mental or strictly physical has done us a great disservice. Labeling it that way has created a false dichotomy. Some view physical illness as something real while mental illness is merely made up or imaginary. We cannot elevate one while dismissing the other. *Because we are embodied beings, illness is illness.* The World Health Organization defines illness as "the ill health the person identifies themselves with, often based on self-reported mental or physical symptoms."[2]

So, are mental illnesses just like physical illnesses? The answer is yes. And the answer is no. Let's begin with the similarities. When we think of physical illness we think of specific diseases like cancer or diabetes, bodily injuries, and the deterioration we associate with aging. Mental disorders are defined differently.

The American Psychiatric Association defines mental illness as "health conditions involving changes in emotion, thinking, or behavior (or a combination of these) . . . associated with distress and/or problems functioning in social, work or family activities."[3] This definition clarifies how physical and mental disorders are the same; both are health conditions. Both arise from within our bodies. The categorization of a physical disorder or a mental disorder is based on the same thing: the symptoms. A disorder is characterized as mental if the symptoms are primarily found in our feeling, thinking, or doing. A disorder is physical if the symptoms arise elsewhere. The difference between a mental illness and a physical illness is in the symptoms, not the source. Both are part of our embodied experience as human beings.

Mental disorders and physical disorders are also the same in another way: opportunity for recovery. One in twenty-five Americans lives with a serious mental illness; one in five of us will experience a mental illness at some point in our lives.[4] The difference between those two numbers is recovery. That means it is not the same one in five people each year. Like many physical health conditions, when treated, recovery is absolutely possible. There are some mental illnesses that have a persistent course, but as with hypertension or type 1 diabetes, with treatment, lifestyle changes, and other interventions, the person living with that condition can still thrive. It's so important for us to recognize that people do recover from mental illness. Mental illness isn't a life sentence, but *untreated* mental illness might be.

> The difference between a mental illness and a physical illness is in the symptoms, not the source.

Perceptions of Mental Illness

I believe that the stigma often associated with mental illness is rooted in the way that we have misunderstood emotions and the heart-mind relationship. If we cling to the disproven misconception that emotion is a sign of weakness—and that feelings are the products of thoughts—then mental illness will continue to be seen as the fruit of a weak mind and a failure to control emotions. But if you've made it this far in the book, you know better. Renewing your mind about the way you perceive emotions should also begin to correct your view of mental illness.

Diagnosis and Treatment

What is the difference between sadness and having clinical depression? Or being afraid and having generalized anxiety disorder? Or experiencing ups and downs and having a bipolar disorder? When a therapist considers whether or not a client has a mental illness, they are considering the intensity of symptoms, length of time those symptoms have been present, and whether they are disruptive to an individual's everyday life.

The *Diagnostic and Statistical Manual of Mental Disorders, Vol. 5* (DSM-5-TR) is a book that contains all of the formally recognized mental and substance use disorders.[5] There are nearly 300 of them, including neurocognitive disorders (like dementia), anorexia, autism spectrum disorders, mood disorders, and more. This section of the chapter provides a brief overview of a few of the most common disorders. This is not to serve as a self-diagnostic tool; however, if you relate to what you read, please do take the next step in setting up an appointment with a therapist to get a professional assessment.

Post-Traumatic Stress Disorder (PTSD)

When people experience or witness a traumatic event or set of circumstances, they may develop post-traumatic stress disorder (PTSD). According to the American Psychiatric Association, harmful or life-threatening situations like "natural disasters, serious accidents, terrorist acts, war/combat, rape/sexual assault, historical trauma, intimate partner violence and bullying"[6] may affect a person's "mental, physical, social, and/or spiritual well-being."[7] Approximately 3.5 percent of US adults have PTSD every year.

Adult symptoms of PTSD include avoiding reminders of the trauma: flashbacks, dreams, distressing thoughts, and other manifestations of re-experiencing the event; being easily startled or reactive; ongoing painful emotions including shame, fear, and anger; and thinking difficulties like concentration struggles and negative thoughts about oneself. These symptoms usually emerge within three months and are severe enough to disrupt life for longer than a month.[8]

Major Depressive Disorder (MDD)

To be diagnosed with MDD, an individual must have five or more symptoms on a list of nine criteria that last for at least a two-week time period. Depressed mood and/or loss of interest and pleasure must be present. Other symptoms may include irritability, significant weight loss or gain without dieting, persistent sleep issues, fatigue or loss of energy nearly every day, feeling worthless or excessive guilt, decreased concentration, and thoughts of suicide.

Generalized Anxiety Disorder (GAD)

It is normal to feel anxious from time to time, especially when experiencing stressful events. However, ongoing, excessive worry that interferes with day-to-day activities and is difficult to manage may be a sign of GAD when it is accompanied by at least three of the following symptoms: restlessness, fatigued more than usual, impaired concentration or feeling like the mind just goes blank, irritability, increased muscle aches or soreness, and difficulty sleeping.

Bipolar Disorders

Bipolar disorders are characterized by episodes of *extreme* mood. Depressive episodes were defined in our description of Major Depressive Disorder. *Manic episodes* are periods of abnormally elevated or irritable mood and high energy, accompanied by extreme behavior that disrupts life. Some manifestations include fast-paced and loud talking, flying from one idea to the next, decreased need for sleep, inflated self-image, excessive spending, hypersexuality, and substance abuse. Individuals diagnosed with *Bipolar I* disorder have experienced a manic episode that lasted for at least seven days. They may have also experienced one or more depressive episodes (each lasting two weeks or longer). Those diagnosed with *Bipolar II* disorder have experienced both manic and depressive episodes, but the manic episodes are shorter and less severe (hypomanic).

Addiction

The DSM-5-TR identifies substance-related addiction with a set of eleven different criteria. How many of those criteria an individual meets determines whether the substance use disorder is mild, moderate, or severe. Some of the criteria include taking the substance in larger amounts or for longer than intended; wanting to cut back but not being successful; cravings and urges to use the desired substance; continuing to use even when it causes problems at work, school, or in relationships; and development of withdrawal symptoms.

There is a specific subset of addictions known as *process* addictions. These are characterized by an overwhelming impulse or urge to engage in a certain *behavior* despite its negative consequences. Common examples of this include shopping, gambling, exercise, sexual activity, and pornography.

Recovering from Mental Illness

The mental disorders you just learned about were described based on the symptoms that are evident when the illness is untreated. Let me again stop to emphasize that mental illness can be treated. People recover. People survive. People go on to thrive.

Therapy

There is no better time to seek out therapy than right now. What I so appreciate about my colleagues is their eagerness to get their hands dirty with their clients to help them navigate seasons in the wilderness. Therapy can help teach you how to tend to the garden within by discovering the past hurts, experiences, and trauma that hinder meaningful connections, pursuing purpose with hope, and building a legacy characterized by love. Therapy is not for mentally ill people. Therapy is for people. All of us can benefit from therapy. For those living with a mental illness, therapy is a critical tool for learning about one's illness, working through the challenges it brings, gaining essential coping skills, and cultivating a healing space nurtured by unconditional professional support.

Medication

There are many tools available for use on our healing journey. One of those tools is medication. Accepting medication to help our bodies function optimally both mentally and physically is not an indicator of weak faith. Consider this: After you break a bone, do you refuse medication? When being put under for surgery, do you reject anesthesia? When you have a headache, do you refuse to take an aspirin? The answer to those questions is probably no. Medication can be a healing agent for mental health as well. When it is included in the treatment process, it isn't meant to replace therapy. It's important to still go to therapy.

Here's the vital message I want you to hear about medication: *God is a healer.* We thank God no matter how He chooses to heal us. We praise God when He miraculously heals us. We praise God for healing through therapy and medication as well. He is the Lord who heals, and we should be ready to embrace every source of healing that He offers.

Bibliotherapy

Reading is not a substitute for treatment if you are living with a mental illness, but it can certainly be a support in your recovery process. Reading books written at the intersection of faith and mental health can also educate those who love and care for someone who is struggling. Here are three books I recommend.

- *The Other Me* by Kandice Ewing is a detailed account of her life as a mental illness survivor. Kandice, a pastor's wife and counselor from Houston, Texas, has lived with the emotional pain of major depressive disorder and survived.
- *When Faith Meets Therapy: Find Hope and a Practical Path to Emotional, Spiritual, and Relational Healing*, written by Grammy-nominated gospel artist Anthony Evans along with media personality and licensed psychotherapist Stacy Kaiser, mixes the power of faith and the practicality of counseling.
- In *The Road to Freedom: Healing from Your Hurts, Hang-ups, and Habits*, pastor Johnny Baker shares his story of recovering from alcoholism. Today he has been ministering in Celebrate Recovery for more than twenty-five years.

A Message About Mental Illness and Faith

In chapter 7 we reflected on the inner war that the apostle Paul vulnerably described in his letter to the church in Rome. He described battles between his mind and his body—battles that he lost on more than one occasion. That is because there are a lot of decisions that we *don't* make about the internal workings of our bodies. Be it the origination, manifestation, awareness, or experience of emotion, the autonomic nervous system (ANS) plays a critical role.[9] When the sympathetic subsystem of the ANS is activated, our bodies can overthrow the conscious choices we would otherwise make. Chemical imbalances in our body and brain can have the same effect. Paul equated this overthrow to being taken captive. A person living with mental illness, especially an untreated one, can be taken captive in a way that you may never understand. Choose compassion over judgment.

When someone tells you they are struggling, believe them. When someone shares that their depression is keeping them in bed all day, believe them. When someone shares *any* painful emotional experience with you, believe them. Validate that what they are experiencing is *real*. Because it is.

To all my sisters and brothers who've lived with mental illness—I see you. Your mental illness is not a personal failure. Your mental illness is not indicative of weak faith. Even if you have been taken captive by post-traumatic stress disorder or depression, know that Jesus experienced the feelings that are part of that diagnosis. He knows how you feel. He is sitting at the right hand of God right now, praying for you from that place of understanding. Even under this pressure, your faith can prevail. Having a mental illness does not cancel out salvation or the healing work of the Holy Spirit.

> **Having a mental illness does not cancel out salvation or the healing work of the Holy Spirit.**

For all of us, whether you have been diagnosed with a mental illness or are just navigating the difficult emotions that are part of the human experience, bring your weakness, your internal battle, and whatever you are carrying in your body to the God of all comfort. We honor the Creator by cultivating our gardens to the best of our ability, but God isn't limited by our limitations! Let Him do what He does best: love you.

That's worth saying again: God loves you. You were created to become the beautiful, unique garden that God has in mind for you. You were made for life. And that's what I want you to walk away with from this chapter. No mental health struggle can ever deactivate the word that God has spoken over your life. It does not exclude you from the worthiness that makes you *you*. God decided to make His home within you. I wonder if sometimes He is just waiting for us to make ourselves at home too—within the very bodies we already have.

Sometimes we're so concerned with being better that we miss the opportunity to bask in His love in the presence of our imperfections. The fact that He loves us *broken* is so much more powerful than if He only loved us perfect. He is too good of a God to ever withhold His love from you. His love has never failed me, and it will never fail you. God loves you. I love you too.

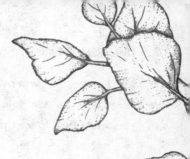

Chapter 10

THE WISDOM OF TREES

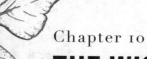

> And he shall be like a tree planted by the rivers of water,
> that bringeth forth his fruit in his season; his leaf also
> shall not wither; and whatsoever he doeth shall prosper.
>
> PSALM 1:3

As we prepare to conclude part 2 of the book, let's take a moment to reflect on how the journey to the garden within began. I saw a neuron that looked like a seedling, then I looked at Scripture and I made a choice. I chose to believe I was seeing the intentional work of God. I believed I had encountered a lesson plan written by the Creator to teach us about how He had designed us to live.

Every time I reflect on that moment in my life in 2007, my faith in God is renewed, because I realize the answer to a question my mother had asked in the 1980s was built into our bodies on the day that humanity was created. Before my sister was born, before my parents ever shed a tear, before my own trauma began—before we ever asked the question—God provided the answer. Please know that is true in your life too! Whatever you are wrestling with right now, whatever pain you may be in, God *knows* the end before the beginning. The Creator is way ahead of you. I promise.

I hope that when you looked at that neuron and that seedling, you saw theology, psychology, and biology collide, and that you, too, decided this must be a God-thing. Don't forget that!

The Role of the Mind in Your Garden

Let's review the analogy that the Creator designed. The soil of your heart is the birthplace and nourisher of the mind. But it's not a simple one-way street. Gardens are complex, interrelated systems. The soil may be the foundation, but any agricultural expert will tell you that soil is dramatically affected by the things that are grown there. Once the plant matures and forms fruit, seeds from that fruit eventually fall onto the soil and take root again. A cycle is established, and when it's a good cycle (healthy plants with strong root systems and good fruit), that's a very good thing! Soil stabilizes plants, but plants stabilize soil in return. The roots help the soil resist erosion because the soil particles are held together by the plant's roots. That means our hearts stabilize our minds and our minds guard our hearts in return.

This insight extends beyond the individual level. Think of us being called by the apostle Paul to come together as the body of Christ, "rooted and grounded in love" (Eph. 3:17). Just as a field of grass or a forest of trees develops an entwined root system that stabilizes the shared soil, humans can come together to have one heart and one mind when we are rooted and grounded in love.

The System Effect

Do you remember the story about my first speech at church in chapter 1? How I was enthusiastically affirmed by our faith community and my father? A seed of belief was sown in that room: *Anita is a good speaker.* Faith and *feelings* flowed through my heart into that seed. It didn't take long for it to swell up and break open. Believing got me *thinking* and asking myself questions.

When can I do that again?

Where else can I speak?

Should I try out for the school play?

Am I old enough for the NAACP's oratory contest?

Why doesn't my school have a debate team?

When I found answers to my questions, I stepped onto new stages and produced fresh *fruit*. The seeds from that fruit fell onto the soil of my heart. A cycle began that has never been broken. I didn't *think* my way into loving to speak. I *felt* my way there. It was a system effect.

Here's another system example that shows how the mind emerges from your garden within. One year a friend of mine was surprised with a beautiful goldendoodle puppy for her birthday. There is a reason why it isn't a good idea to gift a pet to someone who hasn't expressed an explicit desire to raise one. She loved the puppy and did her very best, but within a year she knew she could no longer keep him. My friend traveled for work far too often. So what to do? The thinking began.

Can I return the puppy to the breeder it was purchased from?

Do I personally know anyone who wants a dog?

Might the dog sitter adopt him?

My friend's thinking did *not* include questions like these:

- *How far into the Arizona desert do I need to drive to abandon my dog without being seen?*
- *Shall I take the dog to the parking lot at the grocery store and offer it to strangers until someone says yes?*

Those thoughts never crossed her mind. Why not? They were outside her belief system. Those thoughts could never sprout from the seeds of beliefs within her heart.

My friend returned the dog to its breeder for safe rehoming. She would have felt guilty even considering not doing the right thing.

> ## Your beliefs, thoughts, and actions are nurtured by the soil of your heart.

The first set of thoughts felt responsible. If someone suggested the latter questions, she would have felt offended.

The seed, plant, and fruit are different, but they exist in relationship. They emerge from the system that is you. And all three of them—your beliefs, thoughts, and actions—are nurtured by the soil of your heart.

Spiritual Bypassing

One dangerous misuse of our faith that we often employ to avoid feeling our emotions is called *spiritual bypassing*, a term coined by John Welwood. He was a well-known figure in the field of transpersonal psychology, which focuses broadly on spirituality. After spending years observing his religious community, he defined spiritual bypassing as using spiritual ideas to avoid emotional pain.[1]

Remember the pea plant story? The way the seed grew was by manipulating the conditions. That worked completely fine for our middle school purposes, but we can't grow a full pea harvest using a wet paper towel. Spiritual bypassing is similar. If we don't transplant it into fertile soil and learn how to cultivate a garden, there will be a point at which that plant will wither.

Being too quick to jump to spiritual solutions becomes problematic when we try to rise above the raw and messy side of our humanness. There are two reasons people engage in spiritual bypassing: unfinished business and being uncomfortable with others' emotions.

So many of us have unfinished business in our lives. It's common for us to not want to go back and sift through the messiness. It's easier to bypass, using beloved scriptures like 2 Corinthians 5:17: "Therefore if any man be in Christ, he is a new creature: old things are passed away;

behold, all things have become new." But all things becoming new doesn't mean all things are forgotten. Dealing with that unfinished personal business is messy work. It's like cleaning out the refrigerator and finding those four Tupperware bowls in the back that you'd forgotten and that now contain so much mold you're thinking about throwing the whole thing out. Some of us would rather throw those parts of ourselves out too. Whether you believe it or not, those parts of you are worth redeeming and restoring.

The second reason we do spiritual bypassing is because we are uncomfortable with other people's emotions. Not only do we need to caution against spiritually bypassing our own emotions, we need to train ourselves to stay present with others and not dismiss theirs. When Maria told me about the pain of losing her daughter, I responded by saying nothing, allowing us to sit in silence.

The simple act of being present with someone in pain heals. The best thing you can do when you don't know what to do is simply *listen*. If they are talking to you about their emotions and you're responding to them about their spirit, you're spiritually bypassing their feelings. Meet them where they are. If they're saying they're lonely, meet them in that space. They're trying to connect with you *emotionally*. Be willing to do that. When someone is hurting, we can give them a safe space to talk about where they might be struggling. Just that acceptance can strengthen their faith and may be enough to help them take their next step.

Renewing the Mind

To renew the mind simply means to uproot an existing plant and to grow a new one. While the definition isn't complicated, that doesn't mean it's not hard work. When a plant is pulled out of the ground, the soil is disturbed. Change is emotionally painful. When a new seed is planted in the soil, we need faith and feelings to flow there. We can't renew our minds in isolation from our hearts. How you *feel* shapes the way you think.

Our beliefs, thoughts, and behaviors are inseparable. These are all the seeds, all the plants, and all the fruit growing in the garden within. But remember what the psalmist said about the type of tree we aspire to be: a tree *firmly planted* (and fed) by streams of water. Just as the seed's awakening depends on where it is planted, so does the life of this tree and the fruit it produces.

It's also critical to understand how all our parts work together so that we don't superficially judge other people. We can learn *some* things about people based on what they do, but we must be careful about passing judgment. Scripture says that good trees produce good fruit and corrupt trees produce evil fruit.[2] The problem we have as human beings is that we aren't especially skilled at fruit identification, and to make matters worse, we love doing it. Before Plato ever built his chariot, a desire to apply our own minds to the knowledge of good and evil derailed the course of human history. Back in the garden of Eden, our sister Eve looked directly at the forbidden tree and decided it was a good tree that would make her and her husband wise. She couldn't have been more wrong. Our obsession with the power of our own minds, in the broader culture and in the church, is the deafening echo of the original sin.

A Uniquely Embodied Life

I know that this shift from the mind as our foundation to the heart as our foundation is tough. Trust me, it was hard for me too. My natural temperament is not considered emotionally "sensitive," and my personality profile says I'm best suited for a career in engineering, chemistry, or physics. And I did indeed begin college with a double major in physics and mathematics. I still love science, research, and statistics. So how did I get here, focusing on the roles of the heart and emotions in what it means to be human?

I followed Jesus here.

I still follow Jesus, and I've learned that while no transformative journey is painless, it's much faster if you not only accept but *expect* to end up somewhere surprising.

Your mind is very much the *fruit* of your uniquely embodied life.

We've discovered the relationship between feeling and thinking. We've learned that emotions matter. Hopefully it's becoming increasingly clear to you that your brain's thinking activity is not a "higher function" that stands above and controls your embodied life. Instead, your mind is very much the *fruit* of your uniquely embodied life.

Once again, we see the garden affirmed.

Part 3

THE EMBODIED GARDEN

In part 2 of this book, trees deepened our understanding of the heart-mind relationship. We learned that feelings are bodily experiences that both precede and shape our thoughts and actions. Now, for part 3 we will address these questions: What is the heart-body relationship? How does our emotional health influence our physical health? In pursuit of a powerful life, how can heart-work help us to strengthen our bodies? These answers are in the garden too.

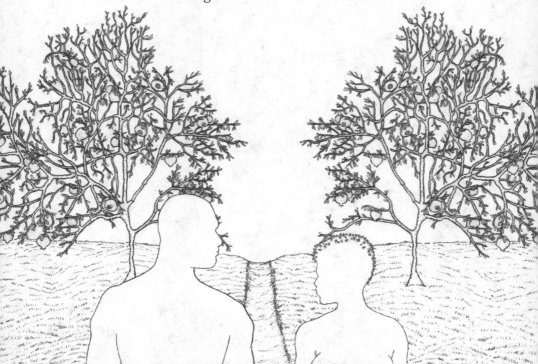

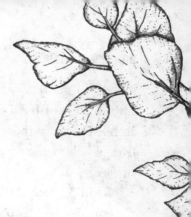

Chapter 11
A TREE IN THE TEMPLE

I am like a green olive tree in the house of God.

PSALM 52:8

The word "begat" appears in the King James Version of the Bible about 140 times. The meaning of that word in the original Hebrew, Greek, and Aramaic is "skip this part." Just kidding! Sort of. But unless you are a theology student, a budding genealogist, or just more spiritually mature than I can ever hope to be, you probably agreed with that definition on some level. If "begat" shows up early in a chapter, there is usually a family tree listing coming. It can go on for generations and is guaranteed to be populated by names most of us don't even try to pronounce in our heads: "and Arphaxad begat Shelah, and Shelah begat Eber" . . . and, oh my goodness.[1] The begats can feel like the least interesting days on anyone's read-the-Bible-in-a-year journey except for one person I know. My father.

My dad loves to study Scripture and believes in the supernatural power of the Word of God. When I was growing up, he often made me laugh by saying, "Keep reading your Bible. God can set you free with the begats!" My father is a Bible scholar. We can easily spend hours talking about the historical times during which Scripture was written and the human perspectives the authors may have held, but he never ceased to remind me that despite sixty-six books being written by dozens of authors across fifteen centuries, the Bible is also just one book with one author and the author is God, so we can—and should—spend our entire lives plumbing the depths of its wisdom and we will still only scratch the surface.

Reading Scripture through the lens of creation leaves me with that feeling. The feeling of being so amazed by what I've learned while still sensing we're just scratching the surface of the depths of the knowledge of God. I hope that you are feeling that way, too, because we are about to dive deeper into the intricacies of how God shaped these fearfully and wonderfully made bodies of ours. We're going to do that by reading the story of how God made the very first human body.

The Body Beautiful

The creation of humanity is first revealed in Genesis 1:26–29. There we read of the Creator's decision to create humanity to reflect the divine image, and some plans and parameters for life in the garden of Eden beginning with the mandate to be fruitful. The first instruction given to humanity in the entire Bible speaks to us as if we were trees. *Be fruitful.* In the second chapter of Genesis, we get a creation "recap" that features the formation of our bodies, and while it doesn't begin with a begat, it is a generational story.

> These are the generations of the heavens and the earth when they were created, in the day that the LORD God made the earth and the heavens. When no bush of the field was yet in the land and no small plant of the field had yet sprung up—for the LORD God had not caused it to rain on the land, and there was no man to work the ground, and a mist was going up from the land and was watering the whole face of the ground—then the LORD God formed the man of dust from the ground and breathed into his nostrils the breath of life, and the man became a

living [creature]. And the LORD God planted a garden in Eden, in the east, and there he put the man whom he had formed. And out of the ground the LORD God made to spring up every tree that is pleasant to the sight and good for food. The tree of life was in the midst of the garden, and the tree of the knowledge of good and evil. A river flowed out of Eden to water the garden, and there it divided and became four rivers. . . . The LORD God took the man and put him in the garden of Eden to work it and keep it. (Gen. 2:4–15 ESV)

This more detailed description of our formation is so special because, of all the things that God could have chosen to emphasize about our creation, this passage centers on our bodies. The body was clearly and intentionally fashioned by God, and it's important that we hold on to that reality. Like emotion, our beliefs about the body are heavily influenced by our cultural worldview before we ever encounter a scripture. Remember Plato's chariot? The dark, ugly, slow, irrational horse was also linked to the body. Like emotion, in Western culture the body is often seen as problematic, untrustworthy, and disposable, but from Genesis to Revelation, we see that our bodies matter to God. While we are living souls on this earth, Jesus wants us to have an abundant life *in our bodies*. The garden within helps us to understand how.

The body was clearly and intentionally fashioned by God, and it's important that we hold on to that reality.

A Treasure Map

Genesis 2:4–15 maps the garden within in more detail than you might think! The Creator planted the Tree of Life in Eden's garden. By sin, it escaped us. A Tree of Life yet stands in His heavenly garden. By grace, it awaits us. But today, right now, a tree of life stands ready to bear the fruit

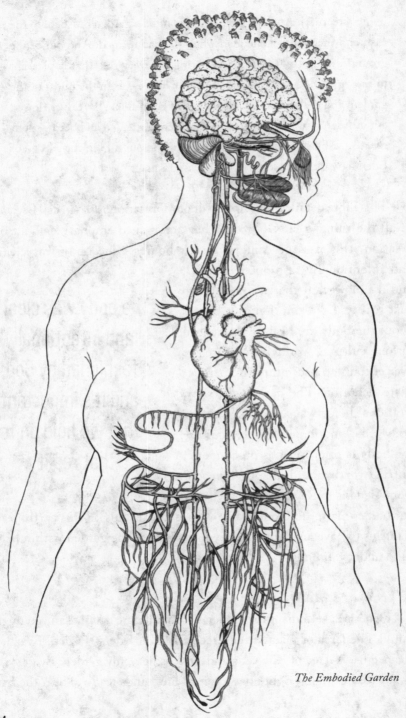

The Embodied Garden

of the abundant life that Jesus desires for us to live. Look at this illustration that I call "The Embodied Garden." It's a drawing of a portion of our nervous system that is linked to our heart, our brain, and our belly. It looks like a tree. The Creator planted that tree of life in the midst of your garden within. To understand this tree, and the role it plays in the relationship between our emotional and physical well-being, let's trace its growth.

The Heart

We must start with fertile soil. Imagine this tree from its beginning as a seed planted in your heart. Your heart is a good place to plant seeds because a powerful underground river rich with life-sustaining oxygen flows from your lungs into your heart. This river is so mighty that, when it flows out of your heart, it uses the largest blood vessel in your entire body, the aorta. The aorta rises from the center of the top of the heart and then bends like a horseshoe. Look at it closely. Do you see the *four* smaller arteries branching off? Once you have seen them, recall Genesis 2:10: "A river flowed out of Eden to water the garden, and there it divided and became four rivers"(ESV).

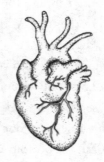

The river that watered God's garden flowed into four separate rivers *after it left* the garden that God had planted eastward in Eden. Raise your left arm. That is the "east" side of your body. Your heart sits eastward in your chest. X marks the spot! A map of Eden within us locates the garden of God within our hearts, and its steady beat calls our attention to that sacred place every minute of every day of our lives. What stronger message could the Creator send us? The place where God first communed with humanity is there, and it's there that God wants to commune with you directly. Your heart contains the holy of holies in the temple that Scripture says your body is.

How incredible is that? But I can hear the questions you might have.

How can my body be a temple if there is a tree in the middle of it? So is my body a garden or is it a temple?

The answer is both. In 1 Corinthians 3:9, Paul said that "you are God's field. You are God's building" (NLT). Psalm 92:12–13 gives us an even clearer picture: "But the godly will flourish like palm trees and grow strong like the cedars of Lebanon. For they are transplanted to the LORD's own house. They flourish in the courts of our God" (NLT). So feel free to describe yourself the way King David did: "a green olive tree in the house of God" (Psalm 52:8).

The Heart-Body Relationship

Let's take a closer look at the way your heart relates to the rest of your body.

Your Root System

When a seed is planted, the first sign of life is its primary root pushing through the seed wall. It grows downward to find water and to anchor the tree. As the roots of this inner tree widen and descend within you, they connect to nearly every major organ in your body and continue until reaching into your belly. This tree in your temple is deeply rooted.

This root system draws nutrients and information from deep within and sends it through the tree all the way up to your brain. It's a two-way communication loop; the brain also sends information back down to the gut, but the bottom-up information flow is much heavier. Eighty percent of the information flows from the body up to the brain; only twenty percent flows down from the brain. I call it our root system, but it's more widely known as the gut-brain axis.

Your Fruit System

Now let's look at the top of the tree. Soon after the seed's primary root is on its way, a shoot emerges, growing upward from the heart where it was planted. The top of the tree is where all the action we want to see happens. I call the upper portion of this tree, which encompasses both your heart and your brain, the fruit system. This is where the heart-brain connection plays out.

Your heart is an organ with its own independent "brain." The intracardiac nervous system (ICNS) is a network of 40,000 neurons discovered in the heart in 1991.[2] ICNS signals travel from the heart to parts of the brain that are related to both emotion *and* cognition, including an organ called the amygdala, which plays a significant role in learning and memory by attaching emotional significance to events. Despite our long-standing focus on the brain, our feelings and thoughts are inextricably linked to neuronal and chemical processes in our biological hearts.

Our fruit system also influences our connection with others. The nerve forming this tree links our heart to our face, our ears, and our voices.[3] When our heart rate is calm and we are breathing freely, we are able to take in the faces of our friends and loved ones. We tune out distractions and enjoy the flow of their words with uninterrupted attention.[4] This state of heart-at-rest supports your cardiac well-being, too, including good heart health and regulated blood pressure.

The Fruit

Before we move on from our discussion of the fruit system, it should not be lost on us that our brain actually looks like a big fruit sitting on the top of our tree. I think that the brain resembles both a fleshy fruit and a dry fruit at the same time. Some fleshy fruits, like oranges or grapefruits, are naturally segmented so they easily break into equal-sized pieces. If you could go to a lab and hold a real brain in your hands (and you weren't too grossed out!), you would see that it is segmented into two equally sized pieces that we sometimes call the left brain and the right brain. And just like a fleshy fruit, when you break it open you would find seeds in the center of your brain-fruit. They are called *nuclei*. Each one is a control center for a specific nervous system function or set of functions.

But it gets better! The word *nucleus* is a Latin term for the seed inside a fruit. Amazing!

But the brain is also similar to a dry fruit. Dry fruits don't have that fleshy, juicy part. Some nut trees fall into this category. Walnuts are the perfect example. The nut that we eat is actually a large edible seed encased in the center of the hard shell that is the walnut fruit. Have you ever noticed how much a brain looks like a walnut?

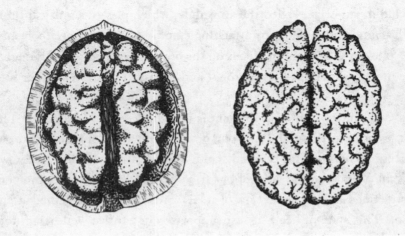

Left: Walnut; Right: Human Brain

And eating walnuts is great for brain health. They are packed with an essential fatty acid called omega-3 that helps the brain transmit signals more efficiently, which supports physical and mental health. The walnut on trees is good for the walnut in your head.

I love the Creator.

The Vagus Nerve

As a spirit-led woman, as soon as I saw this tree, I knew it was worth learning about. Neurobiologists call this tree in the center of our garden within the *vagus nerve*. It's the longest nerve in the body and the main nerve in our parasympathetic nervous system (PNS). The hope, joy, love, safety, and connection that we experience when the PNS activates is powered by the vagus nerve.

The vagus nerve also works to regulate life-sustaining processes including breathing, heart rate and blood pressure, body temperature, digestion, body fluids (sweat, saliva, tears), waste elimination, and reproductive behavior.[5] This nerve heals and supports both our emotional well-being and our physical well-being. The vagus nerve is a tree of life planted in your heart to flourish in the center of your garden within.

Our Embodied Life

Because emotions are bodily experiences, changes in our physical state have a predictable, and sometimes immediate, influence on our mood. Our body gives us direct access to our emotional life, so as a therapist I've embraced a somatically oriented approach to well-being. *Somatic* simply means "of the body." For me, it is a direct translation from my biblical understanding to my profession, yet it applies to every human being because we all live in a body!

As a professional practice, somatic approaches to emotional resilience and healing begin by tuning into the bodily sensations we experience when we encounter any situation. We call this process *interoception*. This is what you have been doing as you have utilized the body awareness tool that you received in chapter 5: paying attention to what you are noticing in your body in the present moment. Maybe you have noticed lightness, discomfort, unrest, tension, or butterflies. Interoception is bringing awareness to one's internal bodily state. It plays an integral role in our ability to integrate and regulate our emotional experiences rather than warring against them. Interoception is the work of the vagus nerve.[6]

The idea of working within the body, rather than the mind, first gained recognition in the mental health profession during the mid-twentieth century, but no modern psychologist can be credited with "discovering" this reality. In many cultures, embodied emotion is a foregone conclusion. It's not talked about or named. It just is. Preclassical Greek culture, Indigenous American cultures, and some Asian languages are known for characterizing experiences labeled as emotions in English as *embodied experiences*.

For example, Dr. Vivian Dzokoto, a researcher at Virginia Commonwealth University, studied emotion-related terms in two indigenous West African languages. In both languages she found that English emotion words could only be translated using the body. For example, fright was "heart-fly," anger was "agitated heart," and sadness was "destruction of the heart." Peace was "heart at rest." In one of the languages there wasn't even a term for the word *emotions*. The closest word they had translated to English as "what one feels or senses inside." That happens to be the exact definition of *interoception*.

The Tree in the Garden

When we consider gardens today, we think of tending beautiful flowers, growing our own vegetables, and producing fresh herbs to flavor our cooking. And that is accurate. However, we often don't think of how trees help gardens to thrive.

First and foremost, trees are good for soil.[7] Below ground, tree roots provide many benefits. They give the soil structure and stability. They provide a framework for the ecosytem to sustain itself. The interconnectednes of your spirit, heart, mind, and body work through your inner root system as well.

Trees also improve the airflow that fertile soil requires. Remember that airflow is to gardens what faith is to our hearts. Furthermore, trees support water drainage so that the soil can get what it needs without being flooded. In the same way, when the tree in the center of our garden within is flourishing, the flow of our emotions regulates.

Finally, trees nourish and replenish the soil. Remember, soil is made of rock particles and organic materials. Trees nourish and replenish by dropping lots of organic material onto the ground.[8] Maybe you are now inspired to go plant a tree in your backyard. I also hope you are inspired to care for this tree already planted within you.

In the beginning, God planted a tree in the center of His perfect garden. When God created the garden within you, He did the same thing. A tree that is designed to thrive. A tree that produces good fruit. A tree that sustains life. The blueprint of God's garden is embodied in *you*. If that system seems tired, worn down, and overgrown, it's okay. God, the Great Gardener, has given us a path to restoration. To restore the embodied garden, take care of the tree. Rest assured in this promise found in Isaiah 51:3:

> For the LORD shall comfort Zion: he will comfort all her waste places; and he will make her wilderness like Eden, and her desert like the garden of the LORD; joy and gladness shall be found therein, thanksgiving, and the voice of melody.

Eden was God's first temple—a place where the voice of the Lord walked and connected with humanity directly. Solomon built a temple for God that echoed the beauty of Eden. The temple had a layout that you may have heard about before. It had an outer court, an inner court, and an especially sacred space deep inside called the holy of holies. As both the garden of God and the temple of the Holy Spirit, when we find

The blueprint of God's garden is embodied in *you*.

ourselves feeling like neither, we can intentionally reenter. God wants to meet with you in the holy of holies that is your heart.

Equipped with this knowledge, over the course of the next three chapters, we will take a closer look at sadness, anger, and fear to understand how the relationship between our emotional and physical well-being manifests in our lives. We will also examine the role of our embodied gardens in engaging our entire system to cultivate emotional well-being and begin living our most powerful lives.

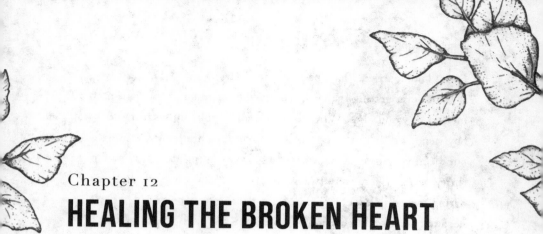

Chapter 12
HEALING THE BROKEN HEART

> They shall come and sing aloud on the height of
> Zion, and they shall be radiant over the goodness
> of the LORD . . . . their life shall be like a watered
> garden, and they shall languish no more.
>
> JEREMIAH 31:12 ESV

Our bodies are wired for connection. When situations disconnect or detach us from people, places, and things we value, the result is sadness. One of the best illustrations for that is when life changed dramatically during the pandemic of 2020. Protecting ourselves from the physical pain of disease exposed us all to social pain, and that came at a steep emotional price. All the loss and disconnection impacted our emotional well-being. The *New York Times* published an article about the effect; the author called the emotion we were collectively feeling *languishing*, and that is a form of sadness.[1]

We are more aware than ever of the impact of grief and loneliness on our spiritual, emotional, mental, and physical health. Yet despite that awareness, the deep lingering pain that sadness brings to our lives can actually discourage us from engaging with and addressing it.

We all have a story with sadness. This is Keshia's story. When I asked Keshia why she decided to come to therapy, she had no problem telling me.

I'm still not married. I have been asking God why but so far, no answer. If I am never getting married, I'm ready to just know that right now instead of wondering. When I got saved, I broke up with my toxic boyfriend. I didn't grow up in church and my childhood was rough, but meeting Jesus changed everything. I was twenty-seven. Now I'm thirty-seven. There were two years of total focus on God, one year dating a worship leader before he came out as gay, two years of "I don't need to be married to live my best life," one year with a guy I met on a Christian dating app who needed that long to hear God say it "wasn't the right time," and three years of trying to let go of marriage and children without letting go of faith. Then there was the one who I was sure was *the one*. He was all the things I prayed for, but I guess he was praying for someone else. He got married less than six months after he broke up with me.

Keshia had staggered into my office bent by the weight of shame. She was ashamed of her deep loneliness and believed she was failing God somehow. Her spiritual practices didn't feel organic anymore. Joy had drained away and, as hope began following suit, she prayed more dutifully and even began reading her Bible out loud so that she could hear the Word and keep her attention focused. She was committed but, week by week, it got harder. She no longer sensed the presence of God in the way that she used to, which deepened her sense of isolation.

Each week she did her best to listen intently to the pastor's sermons and take notes, but she struggled to concentrate. She was in the room listening to her pastor's words, but the sermons weren't penetrating her heart. It was like the words just sort of sat there and then disappeared as if they had been stolen when she wasn't looking. Sadness was permeating every aspect of her life and feeding question after question.

- *Matthew 6:33 says that if I seek first the kingdom, all these things will be added to me, right? So why can't I figure this out? What am I doing wrong? What is wrong with me?*

- *I know I just need to have patience, but I really thought I would be married by now.*
- *I know God gives us the desires of our hearts, but time keeps passing and I still want to have children.*

Did you notice the pattern in her questions? "I know, but . . . I know, but . . ." Keshia was trying to awaken the word-seeds that had shaped her relationship with God, but she was in wayside territory. Her tears had long dried up. There was zero airflow. She finally decided to talk to her pastor and his wife.

Pastor Greene and his wife had long been a steady source of love and encouragement for her. She considered herself an orphan, so they felt like the parents she needed. They invited Keshia to their home for dinner over the following three weeks, to encourage her with love and good food. When Mrs. Greene became concerned about the change she *wasn't* seeing in Keshia, she encouraged her spiritual daughter to add a therapist to her list of trusted voices.

After hearing Keshia's journey, I shared a bit about the different types of grief that might be in her life. She was sad about not yet having the family she hoped for, but she didn't see that as a form of grief. I asked if it would be okay for us to take a few quiet moments to just sit together and honor all her feelings.

"I am sitting with them all day every day," Keshia said. "So yeah, why not?" Her voice was suddenly agitated, as if my suggestion was ridiculous. That double pain layer is personally familiar to me. Sometimes we get mad about being sad.

"I hear you," I said gently. "It sounds like you're doing a lot of that sitting all alone. I would like to sit in it with you so, for a little while, you aren't alone there."

We sat there. In silence. Together.

Keshia didn't say anything, but I saw her body offer up the exhale she didn't know she was waiting for. After a while I asked her to close her eyes and focus on her body.

"When you are ready," I said, "place your hand where the grief is strongest."

She immediately rested her hand against her body as if prepared to finally pledge allegiance to her truth.

"My heart," she said. "My heart feels swollen and heavy. And my chest feels tight, almost like I am struggling to breathe." And I knew that she absolutely was.

What Sadness Does to Your Body

The way that Keshia physically experienced her grief is common. Sadness most often shows up in the body as a heaviness around the heart. Keshia also located her sadness in her chest and her shoulders. The heaviness is at times accompanied by a tightness, making it seem difficult to breathe.

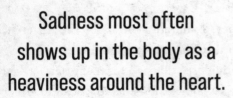

> Sadness most often shows up in the body as a heaviness around the heart.

Sadness literally weighs us down. The weight often feels impossible to shake, leaving our bodies in perpetual fatigue. We slump, move slowly, or maybe not at all.

The Tree of Life Within

Nothing is growing in wayside soil. The ground is barren. In the garden, that translates to the complete absence of the tree of life; we only have the soil. In our bodies that translates to the complete shutdown of the vagus nerve; we only have the heart. That leads us to explore the biology of sadness as it relates to the heart.

Chronic Health Issues

Our emotional well-being and our physical well-being are intertwined. Sometimes we are not aware of our feelings, so it's important to know how unattended emotional pain can affect your body. Sorrow,

146

despair, and depression can show up as appetite changes, fatigue, bone pain, and insomnia. But they can lead to more serious issues like heart disease, stroke, high blood pressure, diabetes, and lower immune function. Heart health is commonly affected because your body responds to depression by reducing blood flow to the heart and producing higher levels of cortisol, which is a stress hormone. Over time, this increases the chances of heart diseases developing.[2]

Digging Into Sadness

Keshia's unattended grief had reached the point of affecting her spiritually, mentally, and physically. It's not uncommon for broken hearts to leave some people of faith feeling spiritually disoriented. We saw that earlier in the book in John's and Lena's struggle and in Maria's life as well. Emotion is an active ingredient in all our relationships, including our relationship with God. When there is a dramatic shift in the way that our spiritual relationship *feels*, things can get much harder. It makes the pain of any challenge so much worse. For Keshia that showed up as worrying that she was sinning in some way that she didn't realize or that God was angry with her.

Keshia's sorrow was also manifesting mentally. She was ashamed of her broken attention during sermons and even forgot her Sunday to volunteer in the children's ministry. Then she gave up on going to church at all after getting overwhelmed just trying to figure out what to wear. She beat herself up for not being faithful, but that's not what I heard. I heard the symptoms of depression. The effects of depression on cognition can include a diminished capacity to think and concentrate, along with short-term memory challenges and difficulty making decisions. I asked Keshia if she was struggling at work in any way, and sure enough, she was having the same issues there: difficulty concentrating and forgetting things she used to easily remember. Keshia also revealed that although things had recently gotten worse, she had been feeling "down" for years.

Soil becomes compacted over time. I grew up in a small, idyllic New

Jersey town called Highland Park. It was a safe place and safer times, so we hardly ever needed our parents to drive us places. We walked everywhere. To get to a favorite local burger place, there was a small park we would all cut through. I am sure that at some point in history there was grass growing where that shortcut was, but I never saw any. Years of heavy foot traffic had worn a hard path right through the grass.

Soil gets compacted under repeated, constant pressure. It can also occur when the soil is too wet for the demand being placed on it. Keshia's compacted soil had been walked on over and over again, trying to hold up underneath a heavy weight for years. She hadn't had the chance to recover from the overwhelm of one loss before life demanded her to move on, only to sustain another loss. On the outside Keshia appeared to be thriving, but she had collapsed on the inside and the soil of her heart was hard and dry. No airflow and no water. Hope had dried up and her faith was suffocating. Keshia was deeply lonely and grieving.

Loneliness and Grief

Of the emotions that sadness can present as, grief and loneliness are the two most dangerous if left unattended month after month, year after year.

Loneliness

Loneliness is not the same as being alone. Loneliness is the emotional and mental discomfort or uneasiness experienced when we perceive ourselves to be alone or otherwise solitary. It is the feeling we experience when our needs for intimacy and companionship go unmet.[3] Loneliness triggers a survival response in our bodies[4] because relationship is a biological need. We need oxygen. We need water. We need food. *And* we need connection to survive. We haven't historically considered emotional pain to be life-threatening but it can be. Prolonged loneliness increases our risk of early death by 26 percent, which makes it as dangerous as smoking fifteen cigarettes per day.[5]

One form of connection that we need is safe, nonsexual touch. There has been fascinating research in recent years showing the effects of how a simple pat on the back or a hug can measurably improve overall well-being. The benefits start from the moment of birth. A review of research found that premature newborns who received three fifteen-minute sessions of touch therapy each day for ten days gained 47 percent more weight than preterm infants who did not receive that touch.[6] In another study, participants who were asked to lie alone in an fMRI brain scanner measured a heightened brain activity in regions associated with threat and stress when responding to a painful blast of white noise. However, participants whose romantic partner stroked their arm while they anticipated the white noise showed no threat reaction at all—touch had completely turned off the threat switch.[7]

The power of safe nonsexual touch cannot be overstated, especially in an era and in cultures where I see it nearly completely absent in so many people's lives. Years ago, a very close friend of mine named Christine lost her mother to colon cancer. She and her mother were extremely close. They lived next door to each other and spent time together every day. Back then, my friend was unmarried and did not have children. A couple of months after her mother's funeral, I traveled to visit her for a weekend in hopes of being some comfort to her in her grief. As soon as I saw her, I threw my arms around her and didn't let go for a long time. She burst into tears. When she sat down on her sofa, she said something I'll never forget. "I just realized that was the first time anyone has touched me in weeks. Maybe since the funeral. My mom hugged me all the time. Now there is no one. I never get to touch anyone."

In the tight embrace of our friendship, Christine's loneliness had dissolved, and in the wake of her words, my touch awareness heightened in a way that has never diminished. I hug my friends. I hold their hands. Sometimes I sit down *right* next to them. I don't want anyone in my circle to spend days going to work, grocery shopping, attending church, going to the gym, heading home, and then doing it all over again while starving for the connection that touch offers. I hope you will now consider doing the same. Hug a friend! Help meet their need (and yours) for emotional intimacy and physical connection. A high-quality twenty-second hug releases oxytocin into your body. Oxytocin calms our sympathetic nervous system, lowers stress, and awakens that tree of life in the center of your inner garden—the vagus nerve.[8]

Grief

Grief is one of the hardest human experiences to endure. Grief is more than an emotion. It's a process and it involves all the big, painful feelings—sadness, anger, and fear. I place it here because sadness tends to be the core and most persistent emotional experience that defines grief. The American Psychological Association defines grief as "the anguish experienced after significant loss, usually the death of a beloved person."[9] The impact that grief has on the body can disrupt one's immune system, contribute to cardiovascular problems, increase inflammation, and cause digestive issues, headaches, dizziness, and mixed-up sleep cycles.[10] Grief can also have profound emotional responses including anxiety attacks, chronic fatigue, and apprehension about the future. It can become life-threatening through forms of self-neglect and suicidal thoughts.[11]

Losing a loved one is certainly one type of grief, but there are other forms that many are not aware of. Thus, we have people grieving right now without even realizing it. Which means there are many people experiencing the symptoms listed earlier without understanding why—the answer could be that their body is grieving. This is why it's important to understand that there is more than one kind of grief.

Grief from Death

In America, school shootings have become a horrifically commonplace occurrence. In 2022, just as the school year was ending, nineteen children and two teachers were killed in Uvalde, Texas, but the ultimate death toll would include one more. The husband of one of the murdered teachers died as well. Joe Garcia had gone to leave flowers at his wife, Irma's, memorial and died right there.[12] His heart was literally broken

HEALING THE BROKEN HEART

by grief. This is more than a metaphor. Mr. Garcia most likely died of takotsubo cardiomyopathy.

Takotsubo cardiomyopathy is a type of heart failure that happens when blood rushes to the left ventricle so quickly that the shape of the heart actually changes. This weakens the heart muscle so that it can't pump blood as efficiently. The heart's newly distorted shape resembles that of a pot that Japanese fishermen use to catch octopuses. *Tako* (octo) + *tsubo* (pot) is where the name comes from. This is caused by extreme emotional distress and is more commonly referred to as broken heart syndrome.[13] Grief can literally break our hearts.

If you have lost a loved one, especially within this last year, and you feel like you should have moved on by now, please be kind to yourself. Grief has no timeline and no predictable stages. If your grief feels too overwhelming, one of the kindest things you can do for yourself is to find connection for the journey. Consider a grief support group or schedule an appointment with a therapist. Neither can replace your loss, but they can provide a space for you to experience connection in a healing way.

Anticipatory Grief

Grieving can occur before death. Anticipatory grief is defined as "sorrow and anxiety experienced by someone who expects a loved one to die within a short period."[14] Adult children caring for ill or aging parents often struggle with this. Your body's response to anticipatory grief is similar to conventional grief—fatigue, suppressed immune system, and lack of appetite. The emotional response can be similar as well, but there is a key feature that is more common with anticipatory grief, and that is the feeling of guilt. You may feel very sad on some days but on other days feel just fine. This dichotomy often leaves many feeling guilt over the shifting emotions. This inability to experience joy in the midst of sadness can impede your ability to grieve well.

Ambiguous Grief

In the spring of 2016, I accompanied my son on multiple "accepted students'" weekends as he weighed the biggest decision of his life so far.

During the opening event at Duke University, the head of the college counseling center said something I still remember.

"Decisions like these are hard. When all the options you are choosing from are incredible opportunities, every yes is also a no. The path chosen is also a path not taken. There is a win and a loss. We celebrate the win but simultaneously grieve the loss."

I loved that moment, because as a mom, I was agonizing with him. It gave Michael permission to make a decision that, although exciting, was tinged with loss—and that was okay. We are allowed to feel more than one thing at a time, and most of the time, we do.

My son ended up choosing Harvard, but not because of the name. When we stepped onto the campus there, he felt a powerful sense of connection. A yes that came from inside of him. I saw it in his body language. That was his place. Michael went on to have a wonderful four years there. The memories are fond, and the friendship bonds remain strong and active. The grief attached to the roads not traveled soon fell away.

That was a form of *ambiguous grief.* For my son it was not life-altering, but ambiguous grief can be incredibly intense and painful. It arises from one of two things: wondering what could have been or wondering if it ever will be. Our capacity to imagine joy when it will only exacerbate pain and our tendency to imagine only pain when joy is still possible is at the crux of ambiguous grief. The death of a child by violence, illness, or miscarriage means that parents watch their child grow up only in their mind's eye, wondering what they would look like now and imagining the beautiful moments they may have had. Keshia's ambiguous grief left her constantly imagining the pain she would experience in life having no husband and no children.

Disenfranchised Grief

"Grief that society limits, does not expect, or may not allow a person to express" is called disenfranchised grief.[15] Examples of this could be the grief experienced by parents of stillborn babies, teachers when they experience a death of a student, or nurses when they lose a patient. It's not that these experiences are uncommon, but since it is often hidden and not talked about as much publicly, it can complicate the grief process even further. When this happens, it has the potential to further disconnect the grieving individual from others and thus impede recovery.

Walking in the Garden

Learning how emotional pain can hurt our bodies is important. It's also important to know that healing can begin in our bodies too. We are a system. I enjoy taking clients on walks through their garden that include their body, their mind, their heart, and their spirit.

When grief, sadness, and loneliness have taken the kind of toll on your life that we saw in Keshia's, it can feel difficult to know where to start. As people of faith, we naturally turn to our spiritual practices first, but that can be hard if you are experiencing the deep sense of disconnection that Keshia was. She was struggling to reach the holy of holies in her heart at the center of her garden within.

When I have clients for whom spirituality is central, I enjoy helping them find their way home to their heart by working from the outside in. We can reenter the garden by first connecting with the body, then walking through the mind to sit down on the soil of the heart in the shade of the tree of life at the center, in the loving presence of the Creator.

Keshia and I did lots of work together during her time as my client. She came to therapy weekly. She helped her body by taking medication for her depression, and we did specific work to heal the trauma her nervous system had suffered. Throughout all that time we also took simple walks through her garden within as she learned to reconnect with herself and God. Here is an example of one of the first walks I led Keshia on—a walk she soon got into the habit of taking on her own. I call this garden walk "Rise Up." Read through the instructions for the entire walk and then try it for yourself.

Step into Your Body

In some emotional states, including deep sadness, our autonomic nervous system isn't in fight or flight. We enter a state of *freeze*. It's as if the roots of our vagus nerve are drying up. Our body can feel shut down. We often experience fatigue and sluggishness that manifest as a heaviness in our limbs—our arms and legs. To return to our window of tolerance, in these moments, we

We don't need to calm down. We need to rise *up*.

don't need to calm down. We need to rise *up*. We can begin that process through our bodies using an exercise I call the 5-R exercise. This exercise will "loosen the soil."

1. **Rest.** Sit down on a chair or bench. Lean forward as far as is comfortable. Lower your head and allow your arms to hang down.
2. **Release.** Inhale through your nose. Exhale through your mouth while releasing a sound that expresses how you feel in that moment. It could be a groan, a sigh, a cry, a yell, or a combination. It can be soft, or it can be loud. Don't hold back. Be authentic.
3. **Reactivate.** While still leaning forward, start moving those tree limbs! Shake your arms, including your hands and shoulders. Bounce your legs. Shake and bounce. Shake and bounce.
4. **Return.** Now, paying attention to your spine, slowly return to the upright position. There are thirty-three bones in your spine, one stacked on top of the other. Sit up slowly as if you are stacking those bones one at a time from your tailbone up to your neck, until you are sitting perfectly upright so that when you open your eyes you will be looking straight ahead.
5. **Rise.** Pressing your feet into the ground, use your ankles and legs to push your body up into a standing position. Rest your hands on your hips. Remain standing.

Step into Your Mind: Testify

Wayside soil is completely dry. There is no water. We need hope. Romans 5:1–5 says,

> Therefore being justified by faith, we have peace with God through our Lord Jesus Christ: by whom also we have access by faith into this grace wherein we stand, and rejoice in hope of the glory of God. And not only so, but we glory in tribulations also: knowing that tribulation worketh patience; and patience, experience; and experience, hope: and hope maketh not ashamed; because the love of God is shed abroad in our hearts by the Holy Ghost which is given unto us.

You may be having a hard time right now, but you have survived 100 percent of your hard days. That verse tells us that we can glean hope from those hard experiences.

I want you to remember a time in the past when God surprised you. Recall a time when He came through in a way that you weren't expecting. As you reflect on that memory, where do you feel it in your body? That feeling is hope. There is some water deep inside you. Place your hand where you feel hope and imagine water coming from inside you and watering you like the mist that rose from the ground in Eden. Now say these words: "Hope rise. Hope rise. Hope rise."

Step into Your Heart

Having found a little hope in this dry moment of your life, I want you to step into your heart. What are you feeling? More importantly, what do you need? Don't move too fast. If you don't know what you need right away, wait quietly. The words may rise from your heart. What do you need? One of the most special things about being in the garden of God is that we can be naked there. Naked and unashamed. Sometimes talking about what we need makes us feel naked and vulnerable, but it's okay to do that here. *What do you need?*

Rest in the Presence

Each garden walk ends the same way: here in the Creator's presence.

Hebrews 4:15 says that we have a high priest who can be touched with the feeling of our infirmities. That word *infirmities* means weakness. We all have human weakness, and it is in the space of our weakness that we have our needs. Hebrews 4:16 says, "Let us therefore come boldly unto the throne of grace, that we may obtain mercy, and find grace to help in time of need." Now that you have been honest about what you need, I invite you to stand boldly in front of that throne of grace in the presence of your Creator.

When we imagine ourselves in the presence of God, we often feel like we have to start talking. Before you do, just be with God and breathe. Remember, fertile soil breathes. Faith is the air we breathe. Let the Creator revive your heart with the breath of life. Let God resuscitate you.

Imagining God's breath filling your lungs, I would like you to breathe in through your nose, 1–2–3–4, and then, as if blowing up a balloon, exhale through your mouth slowly for 1–2–3–4–5–6–7–8. Do this at least three times as your awareness of the Creator's presence becomes more and more palpable. When you are ready, talk to your Creator about what you need. And if that's too hard, you don't have to say anything. Because our God knows what we need before we ask. You can just stand there in His presence with your need laying on the surface of your heart.

Restoring Relationship

All of us experience sadness. You may be well acquainted with loneliness and grief. As therapist and *New York Times* bestselling author Nedra Glover Tawwab said, "Grief isn't always the reaction to a loss of life. Grief is a reaction to loss."[16] Whatever was lost, we know that disconnection craves connection. Now that we have walked into our garden and found a little hope and a little faith, let's begin restoring our relationship zone. I want to see you flourishing again. A first step that we can all take is to let our loss be someone else's gain. The tree of life in the center of our garden flourishes when we care for others. In her book *Bittersweet*, author Susan Cain explains it beautifully:

When we [witness] suffering, our vagus nerve makes us care. If you see a photo of a man wincing in pain, or a child weeping for her dying grandmother, your vagus nerve will fire. . . . People [are] more likely to cooperate with others and to have strong friendships. They're more likely to . . . intervene when they see someone being bullied, or to give up recess to tutor a classmate who is struggling with math. . . .

Our impulse to respond to other beings' sadness sits in the same location as our need to breathe, digest food, reproduce and protect our babies; In the same place as our desire to be rewarded and to enjoy life's pleasures. They tell us . . . that "caring is right at the heart of human existence." Sadness is about caring. And the mother of sadness is compassion.[17]

Relationships heal. Connections heal. For many people, relationships and connection don't feel immediately available, but there is one type of relationship that we can always find: community. Let your sadness reflect the good heart of its mother, compassion. What need would you like to meet for someone else? What gift can you offer? What community are you a part of that you would like to serve?

Sadness is an inevitable part of life, but we can take advantage of the best of it just by embracing the hope that we can make someone else's life better. I encourage you to find a community to serve, on purpose. Put the wet clay of your heartache in the hand of the Ultimate Potter. Allow Him to shape your pain into a blessing for someone else.

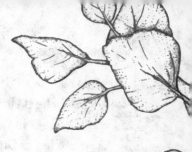

Chapter 13

FREEING THE ANGRY HEART

This hope will not lead to disappointment.

ROMANS 5:5 NLT

Early in my career I led therapy groups for adults who had experienced sexual abuse. Michelle was a group member who became a peer leader. She had grown tremendously after her work in the group, and she had shared her secret with many people, including her family. Michelle's sexual abuse was no longer a secret. Her abuser, her stepfather, had died some years earlier, and he had two children with her mother.

While attending a family reunion, Michelle was surprised by the arrival of her half sister since the reunion wasn't for her side of the family. During the event, people had an opportunity to write the names of loved ones who had passed away on a poster board for their great-grandmother to keep. Michelle was shocked when her half sister wrote her father's name— the name of Michelle's abuser—on the memorial board in her presence. The name was followed by the words, "Forever alive in my heart."

You can imagine how angry Michelle felt, yet she didn't let her anger show. She swallowed it, keeping her face straight and not saying a word. She didn't want to ruin this moment for her great-grandmother.

After telling me this story, I asked if she had confronted her half sister after they were no longer in their great-grandmother's presence, but her answer was no. She had chosen to hold her anger in. Weeks later, I asked Michelle if she still felt angry. She said she was no longer angry and was leaving it in the past. I challenged her.

"Anger releases mighty energy in our system," I said. "It doesn't go away just like that."

I asked if she would mind revisiting it with me, and she agreed. After she recalled the scene and let herself go back there for a moment, she told me how she was feeling.

"Yeah, I'm really mad," she admitted.

"What would you have liked to have done after this happened?"

"I would have asked my half sister why she did something like that."

I nodded. "How did you feel?"

"I felt disrespected," Michelle said.

"How else did you feel?"

"Like I didn't matter," she answered. "She knows what her father did to me, and she celebrated him in front of me. That says to me I don't matter."

I listened to the rest of her story and asked her what she needed.

"To feel like I matter," Michelle said.

"We can't make your half sister feel that you matter. So what can you ask for that she can give you?"

"I can ask for her to respect me. I need to feel respected."

We discussed whether she would go back and communicate with her half sister how she felt and what she expected in the future. Michelle decided to set a boundary; she understood that this was her half sister's father, but she asked that she respect her by not bringing him up in her presence.

"Don't tell all these great stories about him, celebrating him as if he hadn't abused me."

After Michelle told me about this, I asked her what she would do if her half sister didn't honor her request. A boundary without a consequence is not a boundary; it's a preference.

"So if she brings up your stepfather in your presence, what will be your next move?" I asked. "Will you decide to leave? Will you say that you won't attend family events anymore? What will you do?"

"Well, if she brings him up, *I'll* bring him up. If she wants to talk about who he was, *I'll* talk about who he was."

"That's a pretty high incentive," I said. "Are you going to let her know that?"

Michelle said yes. She sent her half sister an email letting her know what her response would be if her stepfather's name was celebrated in her presence. Michelle never received a response, but she still knew her half sister had read her message.

Anger in. Anger out.

Michelle felt so much better after this. This was really important for her because it gave her the opportunity to resist falling back into an old pattern, one where we don't talk about the sex abuse. Where we don't ever bring up our pain. The pattern of thinking that says, *I'm responsible for keeping this secret, and I can allow other people to be more comfortable than me.* A pattern that's not good for her, especially since one thing Michelle wants to do is help meet the needs of other sex abuse survivors. She has already done this in many ways; she's led the group and she's shared her story at retreats and events. Michelle has been living on purpose in this area of her life. She wants to meet this need, so how can she continue to do it?

The gift of her story. The gift of her voice.

If Michelle had allowed her anger to be turned inward, it would have silenced her and undermined the way she wanted to live on purpose. It would diminish her capacity to offer her story and her voice to the community of people who have survived sex abuse. Anger was challenging her purpose, yet she reclaimed her voice. I was happy to see her do this. Michelle has big plans for the coming years for continuing to use her voice.

Anger is always better *out* than *in*.

What Anger Does to Your Body

Anger is not a rare experience for me. Like Cain, Moses, Peter, Jonah, and some of you, my anger is what we therapists call "easily accessible." I know that anger is as much a physical experience as an emotional one. But that's not true for everyone. Some personalities are far less prone to anger, and other people are just uncomfortable with it. They may have grown up in an environment where anger was threatening. Then there are those who learned early on that anger was unacceptable or dangerous. That can lead to repressing anger for so long that you can be angry without being aware of it.

I have a friend who thought that might be her, so she asked me how she could know whether she was angry. In case you need that answer, too, here's what I asked her to do: Think of a time in your life when you know without a shadow of a doubt that you were mad (even if you have to go all the way back in time to that elementary-school boundary violation involving a certain box of crayons). Close your eyes and replay the scene. Really step into that moment. Then notice what's happening to and in your body. Some people notice their face or the back of their neck gets hot. Others may fold their hand into a fist. Anger often involves the sensation of heat and muscle tension. What are you noticing? Learning how anger shows up in your body will help you to acknowledge and process it rather than ignoring or repressing it. Just because you don't feel it doesn't mean it's no longer there.

Throughout this journey we have taken our direction from Scripture and creation. In Jonah's story and in the parable of the sower, anger directly affected the plant's root system. In stony soil, a plant grows until the roots are compromised. In our garden, that translates to the roots of the tree. In our bodies, that translates to the roots of the vagus nerve, so we will explore the biology of anger (and joy) as it relates to the contribution of the gut-brain axis to understand one route by which sustained anger undermines our physical well-being.

The Tree of Life Within

In chapter 11, you learned the vagus nerve forms a tree in the center of your embodied garden. It has a fruit system (above the heart) and a root system (below the heart). Look at it again. From the seed planted in your heart, its roots descend deep into your belly.

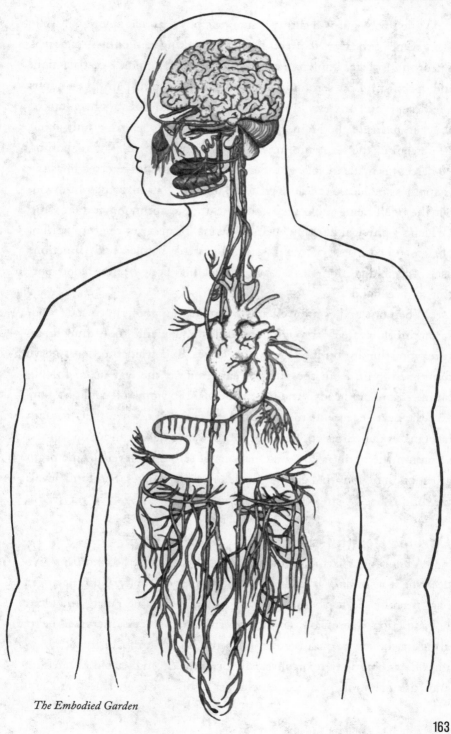

The Embodied Garden

When your gut is healthy, it supports physical *and* emotional well-being. One of the ways it affects both is by making serotonin. *Serotonin* is a neurotransmitter known to support feelings of happiness, satisfaction, and optimism. Low serotonin is a contributor to some painful emotions like despair and anxiety. Since serotonin has almost always been talked about in terms of the brain, it may surprise you to hear that only about 10 percent of the serotonin in your body is made there. The remaining 90 percent is made in your gut. Serotonin is sometimes referred to as the "happiness molecule" because its claim to fame is its influence on mood, but the "well-being molecule" would be a more apt moniker. Serotonin influences physical health by being essential to many of the functions of our embodied lives. "Serotonin plays a key role in such body functions as . . . sleep, digestion, nausea, wound healing, bone health, blood clotting and sexual desire."[1]

When our bodies are well and we are eating good, nutritious food, serotonin flows freely through our gut. Just as a plant's roots draw moisture from the soil up into the stems, leaves, and fruit, the vagus nerve draws serotonin from the gut and carries it all the way up to the big brain-fruit in our heads. And just as the plant in stony soil could not survive the heat because its roots could not draw water, when the serotonin level in our gut "dries up," the roots of the vagus nerve cannot deliver the serotonin the brain needs. Fluctuations of serotonin levels in the brain affect brain regions that enable people to regulate anger. Serotonin levels are diminished by stress and lack of food.[2]

Chronic Health Issues

When anger is too frequent, too intense, and too enduring, we describe it as *chronic*. It leads to problems for your body. Chronic anger has "been linked to obesity, low self-esteem, migraines, drug and alcohol addiction, depression, sexual performance problems, increased heart attack risk, lower-quality relationships, higher probability of abusing others emotionally or physically or both . . . higher blood pressure and [risk of] stroke. . . . Chronic anger also leads to increased anxiety, insomnia, mental or brain fog and fatigue. . . . And it can reduce the immune system's ability to fend off threats, leading to an increased risk of infection, and even possibly cancer."[3] Chronic anger "has [also] been associated with increased pain perception."[4]

All Anger Is Not Created Equal

Ephesians 4:26 says, "Be ye angry, and sin not." Considering the spiritually, mentally, and physically destructive potential of anger, why doesn't the scripture say, "Do not be angry so you won't sin"? Is anger ever a good thing? The answer is yes, sometimes it is. Anger is not a sin. No emotion is a sin. So why this warning about anger and not sadness or fear? I believe it's a question of valence. Let me explain. One way to study emotions through an academic lens is to categorize them in ways that clarify similarities and differences. Two common categories are called valence and motivational direction.

Valence labels emotions as positive or negative. I don't like that because all emotions can play a functional role, so let's say that an emotion is painful or pleasurable, or that it is desirable or not so much. *Motivational direction* refers to whether an emotion is approach-related or avoidance-related. Does it move you toward that something, or would you rather run away? Approach-related emotions are generally pleasurable while emotions that motivate us to avoid or fight against something generally have—you guessed it—a painful valence.

> **Anger is not a sin. No emotion is a sin.**

When something makes us sad or afraid, our reflex is to run away from it or fight until we are safe again. Anger breaks those rules. Anger is painful and highly approach-oriented. In fact, "according to the motivational direction theory, anger is similar to arousing positive emotions . . . and should be associated with approach tendencies."[5] Sadness and fear play defense, but anger plays offense, so angry feelings are much more likely to result in a regrettable act than other emotions.

So "be ye angry, and sin not" makes a lot of sense. Anger makes us more vulnerable to behaving in ways that contradict the values we normally adhere to, but anger itself is not wrong to feel. And not all anger is created equal. We defined *emotion* as the impact a situation has on our body and brain. When it comes to different types of anger, it's especially important to consider the situation. Two situations that evoke healthy anger are boundary violations and injustice. These situations make us angry because something valuable has been treated as "less than." Anger draws our attention to what's important to us.

Boundary Violations

Boundaries are expectations that make us feel safe in relationships. All relationships have boundaries. If you tell your best friend something in confidence and he posts it on social media, that's a boundary violation. If a therapist initiates a romantic relationship with a client, that is a license-threatening boundary violation outlined in our code of ethics. If I hate you in my heart, whether I admit it or not, that violates a boundary in my relationship with God. When you find yourself irritable, annoyed, frustrated, or furious in a relationship of any kind, consider whether it's a signal that an interpersonal boundary has been violated. Michelle's half sister committed a boundary violation. I don't think anyone would disagree with that; however, Michelle had never articulated the boundary. It's important for you to express your needs and articulate your boundaries in every relationship even if you feel the expectation should go without saying. It doesn't.

Injustice

Injustice is a boundary violation at the systemic and community level of relationship. While interpersonal boundary violations sometimes involve an abuse of power, they don't always have to. But injustice is almost always about an abuse of power, and we do well to get angry about that and to act on behalf of those who are vulnerable. That's different from attacking the oppressor. I don't have room in these pages to explain those nuances, so for now, I will refer you to the writings of Gandhi and Dr. Martin Luther King Jr.

Anger as a Secondary Emotion

Anger is distinct from sadness and fear in that it is, at times, the *secondary* impact of a situation. When that happens, the primary impact is either sadness or fear, but anger shows up quickly to protect us from that pain. For example, someone may be extremely angry about being stood up by a date, but their genuine primary feeling is hurt, rejection, or shame. I get it. I would rather be angry than hurt and rejected. Anger can protect us from sadness in the moment, but it doesn't solve the underlying pain. That will still need to be walked through.

Other times anger shows up to protect us from fear. Fear is most often the impact of situations that pose a threat. So is anger, so let's clarify the difference. Anger is most often the response when we feel a sense of both certainty about and individual control in the situation. We know what's happening and feel empowered to do something about it. When the situation is uncertain, and it seems that control is not in our hands, the impact of the threat will most likely be fear instead of anger. Anger says, "They stole my lunch money [certainty] and I'm going to take it back [empowered]." Fear says, "What if that bully steals my lunch money today [uncertainty]? And if they do, I can't stop them [not empowered]."

Feeling both uncertain and powerless is summed up in 1 John 4:18, which says that "fear hath torment." If you have ever been afraid, anxious, insecure, panicked, or helpless, then you probably felt that word "torment" hit you in more ways than one. We'll talk more about fear in the next chapter.

Walking in the Garden

Both wayside soil and stony soil are thirsty. Hope is water that awakens belief in our hearts. Hope is that natural spring trickling down the side of a mountain, bubbling to the surface untouched by human hands—that crystal-clear, pure water. Hope is essential to life. It is not a "positive" mindset. Hope, like water, nourishes the soil of our thought-lives, but hope is not positive thinking. Hope is not optimism. Hope is a catalyst. Hope is what possibility *feels* like. Hope flows first: "Now the God of hope fill you with all joy and peace in believing, that ye may abound in hope, through the power of the Holy Ghost" (Rom. 15:13). It's impossible to be both full of joy or full of peace and completely hopeless about the same circumstance at the same time. Hope is the most important emotion because it's the foundation for every other pleasurable emotion *and* it strengthens us in pain. Hope also sustains us so that purpose continues to grow.

Anger arises from sympathetic nervous system activation. It's the fight response. Ignoring your anger or refusing to express your anger does not release your anger. Once the rush of anger energy that the fight system releases into your body flows in, it will stay there if you don't intentionally release it. When it comes to anger, better out than in. This exercise is one way to release anger from your body. I call this garden walk "Firewood." Read through the instructions for the entire walk and then try it for yourself.

Step into Your Body

1. Stand up straight. Position your body as if you are about to chop wood for a fire. Spread your feet apart. Raise your arms above your head and clasp your hands like you are holding the handle of an ax.
2. Now, imagining an upright log in front of you, prepare to bring your arms down hard and fast as if you are chopping that log in half. As you swing your arms down, release a loud sound with

the strength you would need to chop that log! Allow your hands to complete the entire ax-swinging motion—let your hands move between your legs and then return to a standing position. "Chop" as many logs as you need to.

3. Envision yourself throwing all those logs in the fire of your anger. Sit down to watch them burn.

Walk Through Your Mind: Recall Hope

When we are angry, especially when we are angry at some*one*, we tend to attribute poor character to them. It can be hard to be merciful. One thing that helps is to do what Jonah didn't—recall when God has been merciful to us. When we recall His mercies, we receive hope. Lamentations 3:21–22 says, "This I recall to my mind, therefore I have hope. It is of the Lord's mercies that we are not consumed." When has God been merciful to you?

As you sit watching your anger burn away, allow the mercies of God to be a soft rain over you. Let that hope water the dry, stony ground of your heart until you are again a well-watered garden. See it slowly extinguishing the fire of your anger as "the God of hope [fills] you with all joy and peace in believing" (Rom. 15:13).

Sit in Your Heart

Having received hope into this formerly stony moment of your life, reflect on why you were angry. Did someone violate a boundary in your life or someone else's? What action will you take? What boundary will you set?

Rest in the Presence

Each garden walk ends the same way. Here in the Creator's presence.

As noted earlier, Hebrews 4:15 says that we have a high priest who can be touched with the feeling of our infirmities. That word *infirmities* means weakness. We all have human weakness, and it is in the space of our weakness that we have our needs. Hebrews 4:16 says, "Let us therefore come boldly unto the throne of grace, that we may obtain mercy, and find grace to help in time of need." Now that you have been honest about what you need, I invite you to boldly step into the presence of your Creator before the throne of grace. When we imagine ourselves in the presence of God, we often feel like we have to start talking. Before you do, just sit with God and breathe. Remember, fertile soil breathes.

Imagining God's breath filling your lungs, I would like you to breathe in through your nose, 1–2–3–4, and then, as if blowing up a balloon, exhale through your mouth slowly for 1–2–3–4–5–6–7–8. Do this at least three times as your awareness of the Creator's presence becomes more and more palpable. When you are ready, talk to your Creator about what you need. And if that's too hard, you don't have to say anything. Because our God knows what we need before we ask. You can just sit there in His presence with your need laying on the surface of your heart.

A Story from My Own Couch

A conversation about anger naturally raises the topic of forgiveness. Forgiveness is not my strong suit. I made a podcast episode called "The F-Word" to share my whole ugly, sticky, embarrassing, honest story about how I have struggled with unforgiveness over the years. The first time I confronted it spiritually, I was nineteen years old at a college-campus ministry retreat where we were having 5:00 a.m. prayer every morning. One morning the pastor leading the prayer told us to pray about forgiveness and asked us to intentionally forgive anyone that we had not forgiven. I started listing people and saying to myself, *I forgive this person* and *I forgive that person*.

Then someone came to mind, and I was not able to get any words out of my mouth. On that one, out of the abundance of my heart the mouth did *not* speak. I had nothing to say. But I was disturbed by the fact that in the presence of God, I was unable to shift my feelings and thoughts about this person. A few years earlier she and I had been close friends, then she betrayed me. Granted, I had done something wrong, but I was still deeply disappointed by her lack of girl-code loyalty. You will have to listen to the episode to get the whole story.

But my point is this: I ended up going on a three-day fast just to pray for help with forgiving this sister. At the end of the fast, I was able to say "I forgive." I was able to say her name. I felt so good. I was new in my fresh commitment to the Lord and feeling like a spiritual superstar! I was so relieved that I had gotten it done—but I didn't know then just how much God had done.

Later that summer I went to visit my childhood hometown, and while driving through the old neighborhood with a friend in the car, I saw the young woman I had fasted and prayed for help with forgiving. I slammed on the brakes, rolled down the car window (yes, it was that long ago), and said, "Hey! How are you?"

She looked startled, unsure whether something dangerous was about to happen. I didn't understand why she seemed confused. I chatted with her for a moment, asking how she had been and letting her know what I was up to. Then I said a cheerful goodbye and drove away. A couple of blocks later, I slammed on the brakes again. Suddenly, I knew why she had looked so confused. I had seen her without remembering that I had *ever* been angry! In that moment, the incident seemed to have been wiped from my memory.

That was truly a turning point in my relationship with the Lord. Am I saying that all you need to do is fast to forget whatever happened to you that hurt you? No. Imitating how God delivers others is not the way to go. That was something that God led me to do at that time. What I am saying is to use all your tools. I have a number of steps that I engage in to prevent getting angry and help me forgive, because forgiveness is hard for me. I would rather avoid the work. (You'll have to listen to the episode to hear that part too.)

I also use the applications that I have just shared with you when I need to discharge excess anger from my body. Never lay down your spiritual tools. Too often as we come into an understanding of how we are made and how our well-being is optimized through the lens of creation, we stop doing something else spiritual that we were doing. I don't want you to stop using your spiritual weapons to battle for good things. But I do want you to engage your body and go to therapy. Do everything that's available to you that can help.

Prayer is a weapon. Therapy is a strategy.

The Word of God is a weapon. Praise and worship can be used as weapons. Prayer is a weapon. Therapy is a strategy. Physical movement is a strategy. Meditation is a strategy. We have spiritual weapons—they are intangible but powerful. And we have tangible interventions that make excellent strategies. Use your weapons and your strategies.

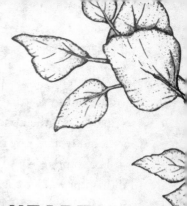

Chapter 14

CALMING THE FEARFUL HEART

> Love has no fear. . . . If we are afraid . . . we
> have not fully experienced his perfect love.
>
> 1 JOHN 4:18 NLT

"I'm not scared."

Even more than with sadness and anger, we often struggle to acknowledge that we are afraid. In part, some of this comes from our childhoods where many of us were taught to "get over it" or simply instructed to ignore it and move on. For others, it can easily be masked by distraction. This often leaves us as adults flailing to know what to do with our fear—so most times we simply don't do anything. I know a lot of people who insist, "I'm not scared." I don't think they're lying; I think they just need help recognizing fear when it shows up.

Have you ever felt nervous or worried? How about helpless, confused, intimidated, or insecure? I guarantee the answer to at least one of those questions is yes. Each of those emotions is a form of fear.

Fear is the impact a threatening situation has on your body and your brain in the absence of certainty and/or control.[1] We all have a story with fear. This is one of mine.

In the townhouse where I lived as a brand-new mom, I saw a mouse for the first time in my life. I was sitting in the kitchen feeding my baby when it ran by. I was not a fan of the experience. For the next two weeks, I continued to see that mouse. Every time I saw it, I refused to go back to that part of the house. Soon I was living in the TV room in our basement, but when I saw it there, I stopped going down to that room as well.

For some reason, I thought I would be safe in my bedroom upstairs. I didn't know mice could climb up and down stairs. They can. One night after I had gone to bed, I woke up hearing this strange scratching sound. Sure enough, when I turned on the light, I saw the tiny creature dart behind the dresser. I panicked, ran out of my bedroom, and joined my sleeping child in his crib. Having seen the mouse upstairs, I felt safe to return to the kitchen the next morning, but there it was. I realized something had to give. I had an unexpected moment of what can only be described as spiritual indignation.

A mouse is chasing me around my own house, I thought to myself.

Then I remembered I had the authority as a child of God and decided I should be able to tell that mouse to leave my home. So I opened the front door (which was across from the kitchen) and, confident that God had given humans dominion over the earth, announced, "I'm a child of God! By the power of Him who speaks to the wind and the waves and commanded the animals to walk two by two into the ark, mouse, I command you to come out and get out of my house!"

Seconds later, the mouse streaked across the kitchen floor, running straight toward the door—and me. I screamed. The mouse froze, turned, and ran back under the refrigerator. After catching my breath, I gathered myself. All I had to do was remain calm. I gave that mouse the exact same command. Seconds later, the mouse streaked across the kitchen floor again, running straight toward the door—and straight toward me. And I screamed. And the mouse froze, turned, and ran back under the refrigerator. I tried one more time. And one more time, the scene played out. After three times, I had had enough. I delivered an alternate mandate.

"By the authority I have in the name of Jesus, go in a wall and die somewhere. I never want to see you again!"

And I never did see it again. I smelled it.

Three days later, I went down to the basement and was greeted by a horrible stench coming from behind a wall in the laundry room. I had no idea what could be causing it. I called a friend to come over and asked what she thought. "Something died in the wall," she said matter-of-factly. "Probably a mouse."

I have had plenty of encounters with fear in my life, but none have taught me the valuable lessons that mouse gave its life for. I learned first-hand that fear and faith *can* exist in the same place at the same time. My faith was not the problem. I had faith in God. I was just afraid of the mouse.

Stick to the Truth

In 2 Timothy 1:7 we find what is probably one of the most oft-quoted (and misquoted) verses in the Bible: "For God hath not given us the spirit of fear; but of power, and of love, and of a sound mind." I want to assure you that I did not face that mouse with a *spirit* of fear. First John 5:6 says that God's Spirit is truth. To have the Spirit of God is to have the truth. To have a spirit of fear would be to embrace fear as truth. I assure you I did not embrace the truth of fear on that day. I embraced power. Fully. I did not have a spirit of fear that day, but I did experience the *emotion* of fear. There is a difference. In other words, I had a bodily response to a threatening situation, which in this case was a four-inch-long mouse that weighed one ounce. Fear is a uniquely human experience. That's why Jesus had to put on a body to know what it felt like. When Jesus experienced what fear felt like in His body, He was having a uniquely human experience, not a spiritual one.

What Fear Does to Your Body

We have an organ in our brain called the *amygdala*. One of its functions is to activate the sympathetic nervous system when fear is present. When the body sends information, the amygdala is activated and redirects energy and focus to facing the perceived threat. During a frightening or stressful situation, people experience the fight-or-flight response we have talked about.[2] When this happens, adrenaline floods the body and causes an increased heart rate, shortness of breath, dilated pupils, and digestive changes, among other things.

The Tree of Life Within

In the parable of the sower, the seeds that fell on thorny ground grew, but those weeds eventually choked the fruit. In thorny ground, a plant grows until the fruit is compromised. In the garden, that translates to the fruit system at the top of the tree. In our bodies, that translates to the upper portion of the vagus nerve. Dr. Stephen Porges's approach to the parasympathetic nervous system views it as having two branches: the dorsal vagal system and the ventral vagal system. The ventral vagal system is also called the social engagement system (SES). I call it the fruit system. When that system is flourishing, we feel open to and connected with others. It's most definitely the opposite of the kind of fears that anxiety brings.

When our tree of life is flourishing, we feel open to and connected with others.

Our SES develops as we are growing up. The more frequent and loving relational experiences we have, especially in our homes and with our caregivers, the better our SES develops. Safe, unconditional love is excellent for our SES. The tree in the center of our garden grows strong and fruitful. If you missed out on that type of environment growing up, it is possible that some form of anxiety is always buzzing in the background of your life, and when a new threat is encountered, your sympathetic nervous system may choke your vagal tree each time. Children who grow up in unsafe emotional environments may as adults realize their bodies are in a constant state of anxious alarm. In his book *Anxiety RX: A New Prescription for Anxiety Relief from the Doctor Who Created It*, Dr. Russell Kennedy explains the sources of that anxiety through the acronym ALARMS: Abandonment, Loss, Abuse, Rejection, Maturing too early, and Shame.[3] Each of those experiences drains love from the life of a child.

Chronic Health Issues

We may try to divide our emotional and physical experiences into separate realms, but our body doesn't do that. When we hold in our emotional pain, our bodies will cry out in other ways. Chronic pain and illness may eventually voice our fear.

Fear can manifest as "headaches turning into migraines, muscle aches turning into fibromyalgia, body aches turning into chronic pain, and difficulty breathing turning into asthma."[4] It can disrupt our sleep/wake cycles and contribute to immune and endocrine system dysfunction. Studies have even connected the prevalence of anxiety and depression to irritable bowel syndrome (IBS).[5]

Pay attention to your body. These symptoms are trying to send you a message about what the soil of your heart is experiencing and can help you know how to best care for it. When we ignore our fears, it creates the very dangers we are trying to avoid. This can create myriad behaviors such as insecurities, people-pleasing, an inability to focus or concentrate due to a constant internal chatter, catastrophizing (seeing problems as bigger than they are), and sometimes even panic attacks.

Walking in the Garden

First John 4:18 and 2 Timothy 2:7 show us that love is an antidote for fear. We can absolutely believe that God loves us, but our experiences with love in human relationships can leave some competing seeds of belief in the soil of our hearts. You can start caring for your own heart right now by making your way to the center of your garden into the embrace of the Creator's love. I call this garden walk "Embody Love."

Step Into Your Body

Since we know that fear is the absence of love, let's begin our walk into our garden by pouring some love on our bodies. Sometimes the best way to love yourself is found in the simplest of forms. Step into your embodied garden by engaging your senses.

- **Sight:** What is something you can look at that makes you smile? Maybe it's a piece of art. A painting. A google search for puppies.
- **Sound:** What sound brings you peace? Maybe it's a song. The sound of waves. The sound of the breeze. Silence.
- **Smell:** What scent calms you? A vanilla candle. A certain lotion. Orange-scented soap. The fresh outdoor air.
- **Touch:** Ask someone for a good hug (at least twenty seconds long). If there is no one around right now, engage your sense of touch in other ways. Run your hands across a fuzzy throw pillow. Wrap yourself in a weighted blanket. Take a bubble bath or hot shower.
- **Taste:** What is something you love the taste of? Maybe it is hot tea or a cup of coffee, a smoothie, or a perfect bite of chocolate. Tickle those taste buds. You have permission.

Walk Through Your Mind

The emotion of fear lives in your body, but we need to pay attention to the spirit of fear too. Remember that Spirit is truth. Fear sometimes offers you a truth that competes with God's truth. Step into your mind and use your attention to turn things around. Philippians 4:8 says, "And now, dear brothers and sisters, one final thing. Fix your thoughts on what is true, and honorable, and right, and pure, and lovely, and admirable. Think about things that are excellent and worthy of praise" (NLT).

The first thing on this list is things that are true. Make a list of evidence that affirms the truth of God's love in your life. The truth of God's love for you. Reflect on what's true and fall into the arms of His love. Once you have your list of what's true, go ahead and make a list of everything else: things that are honorable, right, pure, lovely, and admirable. Everything good points us to the love of God.

Everything good points us to the love of God.

Sit in Your Heart

When we are afraid, we need to feel safe. Safety means different things to different people in different situations. In what way do you need to feel safe? In what way do you need to feel confident? Remember, the goal is not to identify what you need to *happen*. The vulnerability is in knowing what you need to *feel*. Our hope is in God, so we take the need of our heart to God. We trust God to meet the need, even if the method surprises us.

Rest in the Presence

Sometimes we say we trust God even when we're not sure that we do. It can be hard to sit in the presence when you're not sure you're safe there. Not trusting God is the same as being afraid of God. But it's okay to share your fears with the Creator. It's okay to say that you are afraid of what might happen. That you are afraid of what God might allow. It's okay to be honest with God about your fears. You can let Him know that you need to feel safe in His presence. He's big enough to hear that. Sit in His presence and breathe.

Once again, let the Creator revive your heart with the breath of life. Let God resuscitate you. Imagining God's breath filling your lungs, breathe in through your nose, 1–2–3–4, and then, as if blowing up a balloon, exhale through your mouth slowly for 1–2–3–4–5–6–7–8. Do this at least three times as your awareness of the Creator's presence becomes more and more palpable. When you are ready, talk to your Creator about what you need. If that's too hard, you don't have to say anything. Because our God knows what we need before we ask. You can just sit there in His presence with your need laying on the surface of your heart.

Restoring Legacy

I've mentioned the apostle Paul often on our journey together. His legacy has had a tremendous impact on me, and I want to bring another part of his story to the fore. We've explored his human vulnerability and I've shared my beliefs about the battle he described in Romans 7. I believe that Paul's battle was fear-based. I believe that Paul wrestled with anxiety. In 2 Corinthians 12:7 he wrote, "Lest I should be exalted above measure through the abundance of the revelations, there was given to me a thorn in the flesh." That word *flesh* is the same flesh Paul mentioned in Romans 7, and the same flesh that Jesus referred to as weak in the garden of Gethsemane—it's the Greek word *sarx*. There have been many theologians who have speculated on what this thorn could be, and there is no agreement. So I'm going to humbly add my speculation. Because Paul used a thorn as the metaphor for his unnamed affliction, I want you to again travel backward with me all the way to Genesis chapter 3.

In that chapter we witnessed the tragic transformation in Eden. The garden dissolved into the wildlands that we inherited. "And unto Adam [God] said . . . cursed is the ground for thy sake; in sorrow shalt thou eat of it all the days of thy life; *Thorns* also and thistles shall it bring forth to thee; and thou shalt eat the herb of the field" (vv. 17–18, emphasis added). Where fruit trees once thrived, thorns spring up. We are made from that same ground, literally. And when humanity fell there was a change in our bodies. Fear was present.

We see those thorns again in Matthew 13:22, as Jesus interprets the parable of the sower. We know that those thorns are anxious thoughts. We know how tormenting anxious thoughts can be, and we know what anxiety feels like inside of our bodies. These thorns are a metaphor for anxiety, so when Paul said he had a thorn in his side, I think we need to hear that. In fact, the Tyndale Bible translates the word that Paul used for thorn as "unquietness." We all know that the thorns of anxiety are the opposite of quietness in our bodies.

This means so much to me for two reasons. First, Paul's vulnerability reminds us that "do not be anxious" is not the eleventh commandment. It is Paul encouraging us in the same way he likely encouraged himself, even on days when his bodily state choked the fruit of his mind and took him captive. Paul's thorn is a reminder that there is no condemnation for feeling.

The revelation of Paul's thorn also means so much to me because when Jesus gave His life for mine, they pressed a crown of thorns onto His head. A crown of *thorns*! Jesus took anxiety to the cross with Him! So as a woman intimately acquainted with anxiety, seeing that on the cross changed me. Have I had an anxious day since then? Yes. Have I walked from body to mind to heart to spirit to reenter my own garden temple and to dress and keep my own tree of life? Many times. But I find myself outside less often, and I return so much faster because the love of Christ feels so much closer.

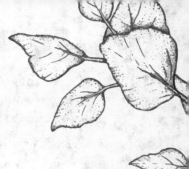

Chapter 15

TENDING YOUR EMBODIED GARDEN

> I will praise thee; for I am fearfully and
> wonderfully made: marvellous are thy works;
> and that my soul knoweth right well.
>
> PSALM 139:14

I ended up giving birth on the hallway floor. It was my fault. The night before, I had prayed for my baby to be born *with no unnecessary medical intervention*. I should have been more specific since God clearly has a sense of humor. An unmedicated birth was my hope. The rug in my apartment was not.

Labor with no meds was an early deliberate decision for me. Shortly after the excitement of finding out I was pregnant with my first child, reality kicked in fast and hard. *I have to actually birth this child? Like, push it out of my body?* The oft-heard belief that labor is unbearable quickly mingled with my fear. A series of helpless thoughts sprang up and would have borne the fruit of inaction had I not called my mother. Ever the Bible teacher, Mom acknowledged that "multiplied" pain in childbirth was among the list of consequences for a certain man and woman having eaten a certain forbidden fruit, but my relationship with Jesus changed that.

"Labor certainly won't be a walk in the park," she said, "but you can kick 'multiplied'[1] to the curb."

When those seeds fell on the soil of my heart, hope and inspiration began to flow. New thoughts began to grow. I decided to take action by learning as much as possible about facilitating this process that my body was designed for. It was 1997. No smartphones. No Google. I was off to the bookstore. Faith and works, my dear. Faith and works.

I found a few books about natural childbirth and fell in love with one. The author explained that an "emotional signpost" accompanied each phase of natural labor and that I could know where I was in the process by being aware of my emotions. This was *not* what I had expected to hear. It went on to say that intense feelings of self-doubt mark the final phase of labor, climaxing in a moment of complete breakdown when you are *sure* that you can't go any further and that you might even die. Once that "snap" moment happens, get ready to push. Insisting that the emotional signposts would be far more accurate than observable measures, the author offered no instruction for avoiding the emotional pain. I had never heard anything like that before, but I've always been an out-of-the-box girl, so I decided to go for it.

With my first kid, things didn't go as planned (surprise, surprise). My son stayed in there way past his due date, so I agreed to be induced. The hospital room, IV lines, beeping monitors, and nurses coming and going made it hard to focus on my feelings. I didn't have an epidural, but still, it was not the experience I really wanted. Looking back, I believed the induction was unnecessary. Thus, my brilliant prayer about medical intervention.

On the day my labor with my daughter began, our doctor had asked us to call every two hours to check in so that she could tell us when to head to the hospital. Each time I told her where I was emotionally, but she only wanted to know about physical signs she considered important: time between contractions, water breaking, and passing the mucus plug (if you don't know what that is, I'll spare you). Other than contractions, none of those things were happening. For the fifth time that day our doctor said, "Anita, you're not close to delivering. Call me again in two hours."

I knew she was wrong, and sure enough, that emotional "snap" moment soon came. I was on my hands and knees in the bathroom convinced that I couldn't take it and wasn't going to make it. Five minutes later I was pushing. My husband called our doctor and did a lot of panicked sitcom-style yelling.

"She's pushing. Do you want us to call you back in two hours now?!"

Then he hung up on her and called 911. Our baby girl fell into her dad's hands before the ambulance ever arrived. There on the hallway floor I breastfed my daughter for the first time. I had never felt so powerful in my life.

Dressing and Keeping the Garden

The truth that our bodies are fearfully and wonderfully made came alive in a new way for me at the birth of Olivia. A seed was planted that day inside my heart, a seed that renewed my mind. Emotional awareness ended up being a better guide than my doctor. Not only were painful emotions part of the process, but they had also reliably affirmed *progress*. I didn't have a war with my emotions. I didn't have a war with my body.

We all have the tools to live our most powerful life. How do we take care of this incredible machine known as our body in order to operate as the garden system we were designed to be? Taking care of it is good for our emotional well-being. Because the body is to the heart what we once thought the mind was, this is the fastest entry point to emotional well-being.

When God created humanity, He made us responsible for the garden of Eden in ways that directly translate to the garden within. Genesis 2:15 says that we are to "dress and keep" the garden. The word used for dress is *abad* and it means to work in or to serve in the garden. Remember, Jesus taught us that our hearts are soil; our bodies were made from that same soil. We should cultivate the ground with the holy reverence that we would bring to ministry endeavors since this is temple work. That also speaks to how we *feel* about the garden.

Even though the fall made the ground unruly and the work much harder, our garden is still a place of value. It's still the place where God wants to meet and talk. Don't let the hard work change the way you feel about the ground. If you do, you may be tempted to go back to war instead of working from a place of peace. Your garden is a beautiful work in progress. It's good, worthy work. Remember, the more fertile the soil, the more air flows and water flows, and the more we are nourished, the more prepared we are to unleash the full power of the seeds we have sown there.

Your powerful life is rooted in fertile soil. Protect the area. That is the second garden responsibility given in Genesis 2:15: to keep. It is the word *shamar* and it means to closely guard or watch over the space. Your emotional well-being must be protected. In doing so, the seeds intentionally sown there are protected. The relationships you cherish, the work of your purpose, and the love legacy you are growing are then also protected. But protection doesn't mean walling the world out.

Protection doesn't mean walling the world out.

Proverbs 4:23 gives us more specific understanding: "Keep your heart with all vigilance, for from it flow the springs of life" (ESV). We are told to keep the garden and keep our hearts. However, the word used there is *natsar*. It also means to guard and watch over, but with a slightly different feel. *Natsar* says to *preserve* something of value. It's not about stopping something from getting in; it's about not allowing something to escape.

Try to keep the seeds of truth in your heart. Do not let your faith escape. Do not let your hope escape. Do not let love escape. But if on a hard day something does slip away, you know how to get it back.

These are spiritual mandates, and we should absolutely engage spiritual practices to live them out. First, spend time in the Word of God.

Like my father said, there is power even in the most mundane parts. I encourage you to memorize passages as well. Worship, God's presence, and prayer are also critical spiritual practices. They are powerful in private and, sometimes even more so, in community. We all know how important those things are.

I wrote this book for Christians to understand why those efforts sometimes become hard and can even feel futile. I wrote this book to help you understand why your emotional well-being is critial to that work.

How to Tend to Your Embodied Garden

Understanding that God intentionally designed our bodies with the capacity to be restored is a reason for hope. I pray that hope will inspire you to take action steps that will help you tend to your embodied garden.

Basic Care

Just like a garden requires daily amounts of water, sun, and nutrients, your embodied garden requires a few basic inputs in order to flourish. You need sleep, water, and food.

Go to bed.

Your body cannot and will not thrive on lack of sleep. Over time, lack of sleep increases your risk of chronic health problems and undermines your emotional well-being. Insufficient sleep leads to an increase in painful emotions and a decrease in pleasurable ones. Being sleep deprived also makes emotional regulation much harder. Sleep quality and quantity is crucial for emotional well-being.[2] Please get some sleep. It's one of the most accessible and most powerful ways to tend to the garden within.

God intentionally designed our bodies with the capacity to be restored.

Hydrate.

Drink. More. Water. A 2021 study conducted on a group of 188 aeronautical military men tested the relationship between hydration and anxiety. Findings revealed that those who were dehydrated had significantly higher anxiety levels compared to those who were hydrated. In another study testing young adults, participants reported feeling calmer immediately after consuming water.[3] Giving your body enough water supports emotional well-being.

Body weight is the main determinant in how much water your body needs each day. The general recommendation is to drink a half ounce to an ounce per pound.[4] There are also helpful hydration calculators online that take other hydration sources and physical activity into account for you.

Don't forget to eat.

Anyone else struggle with this one? When I get super focused on work, I can make it to the end of the day before realizing I haven't eaten. I have had to be intentional about scheduling time to eat. Setting a consistent schedule not only contributes to more stable energy, but your metabolism will be engaged at optimal levels throughout the day, and it can also help manage overeating, bloating, and indigestion.[5]

Eating habits also significantly impact emotional well-being in several ways, including through blood sugar levels, nutrient balance, and the gut-brain connection. Unstable blood sugar levels from eating too little food or too many high-sugar foods can cause mood swings. Adequate nutrient intake supports mood-regulating neurotransmitter production. And a healthy gut fostered by fiber-rich diets is directly linked to improved emotional well-being. As a tip, if this is an area you struggle in, I highly recommend scheduling an appointment with a nutritionist who can help you build a customized eating plan to get your body care on track.

Nurture the Tree

In chapter 11, we learned that the Creator planted a tree of life in the center of your embodied garden. That tree is your vagus nerve. Activating it releases neurotransmitters and hormones that reduce anxiety and promote calmness. *Vagal tone* describes how active and responsive the vagus nerve is. We all want our vagal tone to be high. A high vagal tone means this very important nerve is strong and healthy.

Stress and trauma can weaken vagal tone. Persistent stress can suppress vagal activity and reduce its responsiveness. Traumatic experiences can disrupt the balance of the autonomic nervous system, impairing vagus nerve functioning and contributing to heightened vulnerability to mental health challenges. But just as this tree can be weakened, it can also be strengthened. The garden walks we took together in chapters 12, 13, and 14 each involved the vagus nerve. The deep breathing with slow, extended exhales that conclude each walk activates the vagus nerve and supports vagal tone. The breath of life the Creator first breathed into Adam does so much more than keep us alive. It also helps us thrive!

Improving vagal tone can be achieved in various ways, including some other things we have already discussed. In addition to deep breathing physical exercise, a healthy diet and sufficient sleep can all strengthen your vagus nerve. Spending time in creation is great for your vagus nerve too (of course!). Nature activates the vagus nerve through fresh air, relaxing sounds like bird songs or crashing ocean waves, and the calming effect of the color green. Reducing stress through relaxation exercises or therapy and fostering positive social connections are also important avenues.

As a church kid, so many of our family's social connections revolved around the people who worshipped with us. I doubt many folks in our congregation knew much about the vagus nerve back then, but that doesn't mean we weren't nurturing the tree in the center of our gardens. At least once per Sunday, someone stepped up to the podium and said, "Hug your neighbor!" Hugging and physical touch, especially warm and supportive embraces, have been shown to stimulate the vagus nerve. We also sang together. Singing activates the vagus nerve through deep breathing, muscle engagement in the throat, and the emotional and physiological effects of vocal expression. And in my traditional African

American church, we also danced. A lot. Dancing can strengthen the vagus nerve through bilateral rhythmic movement. I love digging into the biology of it all, but scripture has been directing us from the beginning: "Let them praise his name in the dance: let them sing praises unto him" (Psalm 149:3).

Through this book you have traveled through the gardens of the Bible with me and have allowed me to walk with you through the garden of your own heart. You have learned that your spirit, mind, heart, and body are interdependent on one another as an embodied system. You have moved through the core painful emotions of sadness, anger, and fear, becoming aware of their presence in your body without fearing them so that you can let them flow. You got some dirt underneath your fingernails when you went digging and found weeds that needed to be pulled. You've bravely inhaled faith in a way you likely never have before, allowing the God of hope to propel you toward His perfect love. You are walking the ground of your garden, and the Gardener is so pleased with what He's found. This is purpose-filled work. This is legacy work. This is your work. And this is your powerful life.

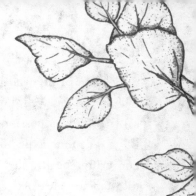

FROM WAR TO PEACE

And God blessed them, and God said unto them, Be fruitful,
and multiply, and replenish the earth, and subdue it: and have
dominion over the fish of the sea, and over the fowl of the air,
and over every living thing that moveth upon the earth.

GENESIS 1:28

People go to therapy for a lot of reasons.

"I have been having nightmares the last few months and they are
intensifying."

"I have been in a lot of physical pain. My doctor can't pinpoint a
cause. Could this be in my head?"

"The amazing guy I have been seeing wants to marry me but I'm not
sure marriage is the right thing for me."

One thing I have not heard is, "I'm here because everything is great
and I'm just wondering if there is more to wellness so that I don't miss a
thing!" That has never happened. Change is usually motivated by pain.
And not a small amount of pain. Once the painful issue is resolved, we
consider the problem solved. But is well-being simply the absence of pain,
or is there more to pursue? From philosophers to public health workers
to psychologists and beyond, there is no single agreed-upon definition
of what it means for human beings to flourish. For me, the spiritual

dimension of my well-being begins with following Jesus. That may be true for you as well, but what about the other parts of us? How does it all fit? Those questions have been at the center of the journey of this book. We found the answer in a garden. And among biblical traditions concerning health, the concept of shalom is the perfect way to summarize all that we've learned.

From Restlessness to Shalom

The Hebrew word *shalom* is often translated as "peace," but that definition alone is too shallow. *Shalom* is more robust than the way that we use the word *peace* in contemporary American English. *Shalom*'s original meaning is "well-being," a well-being that is expansive and relational. Nicholas Wolterstorff, Professor Emeritus of Philosophical Theology at Yale Divinity School, describes shalom as the "Creator's vision for humanity," and goes on to define it as follows:

> Dwelling at peace in all relationships: with God, with himself, with his fellows, with nature, a peace which is not merely the absence of hostility . . . but a peace which at its highest is enjoyment [and to] enjoy these relationships, to see them flourish: with God, through worship and service; with our neighbors, through delighting in justice and community; with nature, through enjoying our physical surroundings in work and play; and, with ourselves, by acknowledging we are created in God's image and for his good pleasure. [1]

Shalom is a vast and beautiful concept. Wolterstorff taught that "at its heart shalom means *flourishing*." I love that word. It means "growing vigorously; thriving; prosperous."[2] It uses the language of plants to describe the type of life we all hope to live. Eden was the Creator's first demonstration of shalom: every relationship in perfect harmony.

The creation account in Genesis sets the stage for the Bible's entire vision of humanity's purpose and destiny, and it reveals a loving and creative God who built a beautifully ordered universe. While the world we live in now is broken and marred in all kinds of ways, it remains fundamentally good—because that's how God originally created it. That original goodness is shalom.

If shalom names the flourishing of a rightly ordered cosmos, it's no surprise that it is also an excellent way of describing the goal of therapy. This book is specifically about ending the war with our emotions in order to unlock a richer and more powerful way of living. Just about any challenge to our emotional or mental health starts as an internal conflict, a disordering of our thoughts and feelings, a war within—in other words, a disruption of shalom. My work as a therapist involves helping people recognize the interdependent system that is their spirit, heart, mind, and body—to discover peaceful balance beyond the brokenness that we all experience.

Finding the Answers in His Word

When we talk about mental and emotional health, and human flourishing more broadly, we shouldn't be surprised that we can look to the shalom of God's original creative work to discover insights about the internal shalom we're cultivating.

You'll recall that this journey to our garden within began at my kitchen table in 2007. It was sparked by a single Bible verse: "For since the creation of the world [God's] invisible attributes are clearly seen, being understood by the things that are made, even His eternal power and Godhead, so that they are without excuse" (Rom. 1:20 NKJV).

I had just begun a Bible study focused on the book of Romans when I was arrested by that verse. My study took an immediate detour straight to Genesis. I slowly reread the first three chapters, trying to absorb each word as if it was my first time seeing and hearing them. Then, instinctively, I walked over to our bookshelves to look for more information.

Which commentary should I search?

Is there a theology book of some kind that covers this?

Where do I go from here?

Standing there in the silence, I listened for an answer. It came. That quiet voice of the Spirit said very clearly, *Just read your Bible.* Instructions don't get much simpler than that, so I obeyed the voice of the Spirit. I just read my Bible. I kept my *Strong's Concordance* close at hand to help me along. That concordance is an index listing every word in the King James Version of the Bible. You can look up "tree" or "seed" or any other word and find a list of all the verses where that word is mentioned. Along the way, I made occasional use of Bible dictionaries as well.

Here is the brilliance of the Creator—I don't need a deep exegesis or an assessment of culture and context during biblical times to know what a tree is. We all know what a tree is.

Leaves, fruit, and water. We all know.

A seed and soil. We all know.

I think that was probably the Creator's point. We all speak the language of creation.

The alignment between Scripture, our bodies, and the plant kingdom astounded me then and I remain in awe today as technological advances and new research allow us to clearly see more and more of what the Creator made. I always believed that the pragmatic answers about mental health, illness, and well-being could be found in this sacred text, but truly, from the moment I saw that neuron for the first time, I have been overwhelmed by what the answers turned out to be. I shouldn't be surprised that those answers flipped the tables of our minds and centered our hearts. I shouldn't be, but I was. I'm so grateful though. Living from the heart is so much better.

I also now understand at least part of the reason why the Spirit told me to *just read my Bible* on this specific journey.

In very recent years, I've read some beautiful theological musings about creation—some by those considered the fathers of the Western church and some newer thinkers as well. I have also read some assertions that could have ended this journey before it ever began. Assertions about what the Bible cannot do and cannot answer. Assertions that insist there is no new knowledge or insight to gain, and that each thing can only mean one thing ever, as if the Creator is not capable of doing many things at once. I for one believe that the Creator is not limited the way we are.

Throughout history, theologians have emphasized the importance of recognizing that creation is itself a sacred text to be read, insisting that "God has presented us with 'two books'—Scripture and the natural world."[3] Saint Augustine (AD 395–430), a North African philosopher considered to be the most important Christian thinker next to the apostle Paul,[4] said this:

> Others, in order to find God, will read a book. Well, as a matter of fact there is a certain great big book, the book of created nature. Look carefully at it top and bottom, observe it, read it. God did not make letters of ink for you to recognize him in; he set before your eyes all these things he has made. Why look for a louder voice?[5]

Reading the book of creation may have been new to you. If so, I hope you have enjoyed it. Reading creation in dialogue with Scripture illuminates both and helps us guard against misreading either one. The key is to stay focused on what we can learn about the Creator. When we explore Scripture just to win an argument or to urgently prove to someone that we are right and they are wrong, it's no longer about God; it's about us. Let's keep searching for what the Creator wrote about Himself in the things that He made, including our bodies. All great painters throughout history have signature elements in their work. A particular stroke of the paintbrush. An identifiable color palette. Unique uses of shadow. The very subjects they paint. These signatures are often so unique that students of art can see a work and immediately identify the painter with no prior knowledge of that piece. Well, when I see you I am looking at the Creator's incredible work of art and I see His signature, clearly.

In His Image: The Power of Words

For centuries, theologians and scholars have struggled to explain how man is made in the image of God. Some argue that we bear the image of God because we are capable of rational thought in a way that animals aren't. Others emphasize power, arguing that we bear the image of God because He gave us dominion. Some even suggest it's our capacity for creativity. Our journey through the gardens of Scripture and the garden within suggests something more: words.

From the garden of Eden, through the garden parables, to the garden of Gethsemane, the Garden Tomb, the garden city, and our garden within, the Creator's words are represented by an imperishable seed. While literal seeds may last hundreds of years, and the impact of human words can last for generations, the Word of the Lord lasts forever. God's Word never passes away and it cannot fail to accomplish what it was dispatched to do. The Creator's Son is Himself a Word who became a seed that was embodied to redeem the world. The power of God's Word is indeed eternal. It cannot pass away.

In many ways humanity is not unique among the creations that occupy the heavens and the earth. Aside from the extensive parallels between plant life and human life, the relationships between us are undeniable. Plants and humans depend on each other to breathe; we co-respire. But humanity has commonalities with the animals as well. We know animals do communicate with each other and a parrot can even imitate the sound of human words, but no other creation possesses the power of language that we do. Why? Because the Creator wanted to have a relationship with us. To walk in the garden in the cool of the day to talk with us. To be His children. We were meant to be part of the family. We see evidence of this in Scripture as well. On the sixth day of creation, after the animals were made, Scripture recounts, "And God said, Let us make man in our image, after our likeness" (Gen. 1:26). The presence of the entire Godhead was significant to us being created in the image of God.

There is only one other time in Scripture when God says "let us." Words are involved then too. It was the Tower of Babel.

> And the whole earth was of one language, and of one speech. And it came to pass, as they journeyed from the east, that they found a plain in the land of Shinar; and they dwelt there. And they said one to another, Go to, *let us* make brick, and burn them thoroughly. And they had brick for stone, and slime had they for morter. And they said, Go to, *let us* build us a city and a tower, whose top may reach unto heaven; and *let us* make us a name, lest we be scattered abroad upon the face of the whole earth. And the LORD came down to see the city and the tower, which the children of men builded. And the Lord said, Behold, the people is one, and they have all one language; and this they begin to do: and now nothing will be restrained from them, which they have imagined to do. Go to, *let us* go down, and there confound their language, that they may not understand one another's speech. So the LORD scattered them abroad from thence upon the face of all the earth: and they left off to build the city. (Gen. 11:1–8, emphasis added)

The Lord himself acknowledged the power the people derived from having one shared language—the capacity to speak and plant by the exchange of words—and one shared heart. They could wield the power of being made in the image of God even though they weren't doing it in a way that pleased God. So the Godhead came and disrupted the unity of their language, but even then, and even now, we retain the image of God within us. Our words are still powerful. Our word-seeds can create and destroy. We must speak carefully. Our power is not the same as God's, but it is a reflection of His power. Words are spiritually powerful. My Bible tells me so.

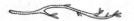

On my nineteenth birthday my father gifted me a leather-bound King James Scofield Study Bible. The same Bible my mom's father had given her. On the first blank page inside, my dad wrote these words:

> Dear Anita,
>> There is no question for which this book does not have the answer.
>>> Love,
>>> Daddy

My dad was right.

Cultivate the soil of your heart and plant powerful word-seeds. Do it with clear intention. Dress and keep your garden within. You were created that way.

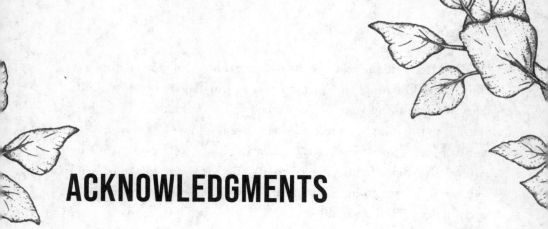

ACKNOWLEDGMENTS

> Dependence starts when we are born and lasts until we die. . . . We mistakenly fall prey to the myth that successful people are those that help rather than need, and broken people need rather than help. . . . But the truth is that no amount of money, influence, resources, or determination will change our physical, emotional, and spiritual dependence on others.
> BRENÉ BROWN, *RISING STRONG*

In the three years preceding the release of *The Garden Within*, I was more acutely aware of my dependence on others than I have ever been. That's because releasing this book into the world is one of the scariest things I have ever done. And as life would have it, this work was incubated and birthed during a long season of turbulence. On many days and many nights, the soil of my own heart was watered by my tears, but I am grateful that I was never in it alone. I was dependent on many people. I want to acknowledge that.

I acknowledge my dependence on my family.

To Dad—thank you for being an example of consistency. Consistent presence. Consistent support. Consistent leadership. Consistent growth. Great is thy faithfulness! You reflect the character of God in that way.

To Mom—thank you for being an example of power and self-knowledge. Growing up watching you inoculated me against limits. Because of you, my view of my capacity as a woman has never been blurred, so my voice has never been sacrificed.

To Mike—thank you for the space you made for me to pursue my calling. To Michael and Olivia—thank you for the privilege of being your mom. I learn so much about life by seeing it through your eyes. I love you deeply and unconditionally.

To Mama and Papa J—better known to others as Bishop T. D. and Lady Serita Jakes, thank you for being spiritual parents. Thank you for seeing me, trusting me, and always pushing me forward.

I acknowledge my dependence on my friends.

I will never know why I have been blessed with the honor of calling such incredible women my friends.

To Tangela, Celeste, and Sarah—thank you for being my inner circle; there are no words for what you mean to me. For the tears and the fears, you are there. For laughter over good food, you are there. In all the joy and through all the pain you assure me that I am connected, valued, and safe. Thank you.

To Mitra, Kendrea, and Danae—our daily lives are separated by many miles, but our hearts are not. Thank you for always answering the call.

To Donna, Holly, and Lisa—thank you for your wisdom, your prayers, and the spiritual insights that brought light during dark segments of the journey.

I acknowledge my dependence on my team.

To Esther Fedorkevich—my literary agent, you personify "above and beyond." Thank you for staunchly believing in the importance of this work and making sure that I kept believing it too. I am forever grateful to you and everyone at the Fedd Agency.

To Daniel Marrs, Brigitta Nortker, John Andrade, Lisa Beech, Andrew Stoddard, and the whole team at Thomas Nelson—thank you for hanging on for a wild, often bumpy, but never boring ride. You have poured your hearts into spreading the message of this book. Daniel, thank you for being my editor. Your gentle brilliance and depth of experience were invaluable to me.

To Woman Evolve, the Chandy Group, and MAC Creative Agency—thank you for embracing me. I deeply respect the way that you serve. Integrity is a superpower.

To Kara Schneider, Nate Pointer, Yana Jenay Connor, Kenneth Hagler II, Billy Stevenson III, Tim Paulson, Jenny Baumgartner, Janet Talbert, and Margot Starbuck—in an official or unofficial capacity, and for varying lengths of time, each of you were a part of my team. Thank you for the good seeds you planted and for the ways that you watered this work.

I acknowledge my dependence on my Creator.

Now to him who is able to keep [me] from stumbling and to present [me] blameless before the presence of his glory with great joy, to the only God, our Savior, through Jesus Christ our Lord, be glory, majesty, dominion, and authority, before all time and now and forever. Amen. (Jude 1:24–25 ESV)

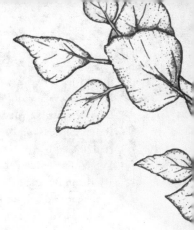
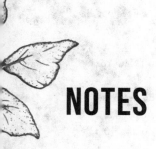

NOTES

Chapter 1: The Seedling

1. Cleveland Clinic, "You Are Your Brain," Healthy Brains, accessed December 20, 2022, https://healthybrains.org/brain-facts/.
2. *The Matrix*, written and directed by Lana Wachowski and Lilly Wachowski, produced by Joel Silver (Burbank, CA: Warner Bros., 1999), DVD.
3. The Editors at Encyclopaedia Britannica, "Rutherford Model," *Encyclopaedia Britannica*, updated May 17, 2023, https://www.britannica.com/science/Rutherford-model.
4. Ali Elhakeem et al., "Aboveground Mechanical Stimuli Affect Belowground Plant-Plant Communication," *PLoS ONE* 13, no. 5 (May 2018): e0195646, https://doi.org/10.1371/journal.pone.0195646.
5. Ramakrishna Akula and Soumya Mukherjee, "New Insights on Neurotransmitters Signaling Mechanisms in Plants," *Plant Signaling & Behavior* 15, no. 6 (May 2020): e1737450, https://doi.org/10.1080/15592324.2020.1737450.
6. See Gen. 2–3; Matt. 13:1–32; 26:36–46; Mark 4:26–29; Luke 22:40–46; John 19:38–42; Rev. 21:22–22:7.

Chapter 2: Check the Flow

1. As with all the stories that I share in the pages of this book, I have changed the names, circumstances, and details to protect the privacy of those involved. Further, some of the stories reflect the shared, repeated patterns of emotional pain, brokenness, and healing that I encounter in my work, rather than being based on any one person's experiences. However, the struggles and insights accurately reflect the journeys of healing that I have had the privilege of guiding people through. The individuals whose journeys I describe in this book have reviewed and approved of the way their stories have been presented.
2. Elizabeth Belfiore, "Dancing with the Gods: The Myth of the Chariot in Plato's

'Phaedrus,'" *American Journal of Philology* 127, no. 2 (Summer 2006): 185–217, https://www.jstor.org/stable/3804910.

3. Simo Knuuttila, "Medieval Theories of the Emotions," Stanford Encyclopedia of Philosophy, last updated June 25, 2022, https://plato.stanford.edu/archives /fall2022/entries/medieval-emotions/.

4. Leonard Mlodinow, *Emotional: How Feelings Shape Our Thinking* (New York: Pantheon Books, 2022), 10.

5. Patrick R. Steffen, Dawson Hedges, and Rebekka Matheson, "The Brain Is Adaptive Not Triune: How the Brain Responds to Threat, Challenge, and Change," *Frontiers in Psychiatry* 13 (April 2022): 802606, https://doi.org/10.3389 /fpsyt.2022.802606.

6. Knuuttila, "Medieval Theories of the Emotions."

7. Forces of Change, "What Is Soil?," Smithsonian Environmental Research Center, accessed April 19, 2023, https://forces.si.edu/soils/02_01_00.html.

8. Elizabeth A. Livingstone and Frank Leslie Cross, eds., *The Oxford Dictionary of the Christian Church* (New York: Oxford University Press), s.v. "heart."

9. Spiros Zhodhiates, *Hebrew-Greek Key Word Study Bible: KJV Edition*, 2nd rev. ed. (Chattanooga, TN: AMG Publishers, 2008), s.v. "heart."

10. Francis Brown, S. R. Driver, and Charles A. Briggs, *A Hebrew and English Lexicon of the Old Testament: With an Appendix Containing the Biblical Aramaic* (Oxford: Clarendon Press, 1966), quoted in New Testament Greek Lexicon: King James Version, s.v. "leb," Bible Study Tools, accessed May 23, 2023, https:// www.biblestudytools.com/lexicons/hebrew/kjv/leb.html.

11. APA Dictionary of Psychology, s.v. "belief," American Psychological Association, accessed December 21, 2022, https://dictionary.apa.org/.

12. *Strong's Concordance*, s.v. "5397. neshamah," Bible Hub, accessed December 21, 2022, https://biblehub.com/hebrew/5397.htm.

13. Christoph Zenzmaier et al., "Response of Salivary Biomarkers to an Empathy Triggering Film Sequence—A Pilot Study," *Scientific Reports* 11 (2021), https:// doi.org/10.1038/s41598-021-95337-4.

14. See Maital Neta and Ingrid J. Haas, "Movere: Characterizing the Role of Emotion and Motivation in Shaping Human Behavior," in Neta and Haas, eds., *Emotion in the Mind and Body*, vol. 66 of Nebraska Symposium on Motivation in Shaping Human Behavior, ed. Lisa Crockett (Cham, Switzerland: Springer Nature, 2019), 1–9, https://doi.org/10.1007/978-3-030-27473-3_1.

Chapter 3: Good Ground and Your Most Powerful Life

1. Paul J. Zinke, *Mediterranean Analogs of California Soil Vegetation Types* (Berkeley: University of California, 1965), https://apps.dtic.mil/sti/citations/AD0643416.

2. Zinke, *Mediterranean Analogs*, 12.

3. Eugene Peterson, *The Pastor: A Memoir* (San Francisco: HarperOne, 2011), 137.

4. Chelsey Luger and Thosh Collins, *The Seven Circles: Indigenous Teachings for Living Well* (San Francisco: HarperOne, 2022), 97–126.
5. Vanessa Bauza, "Finding the Oldest Tree Is Facing Competition: 3 Stories You May Have Missed," Conservation International, June 6, 2022, https://www.conservation.org/blog/the-worldsdiscovery.com/nature/finding-the-oldest-tree-is-facing-competition-3-stories-you-may-have-missed.
6. While she shared this comment in an informal spoken setting, she shared a similar message in an Instagram post: Yana Jenay Conner (@yanajenay), "Who said you had to be married and on your second kid by 32?," Instagram photo, February 9, 2021, https://www.instagram.com/p/CLEv-JlnxaF/?igshid=YmMyMTA2M2Y=.
7. Robert J. Sternberg, "Duplex Theory of Love: Triangular Theory of Love and Theory of Love As a Story," Robert J. Sternberg (website), accessed December 21, 2022, http://www.robertjsternberg.com/love.

Chapter 4: Ground Zero
1. APA Dictionary of Psychology, s.v. "sadness."
2. APA Dictionary of Psychology, s.v. "anger."
3. Antje Schmitt, Michael M. Gielnik, and Sebastian Seibel, "When and How Does Anger During Goal Pursuit Relate to Goal Achievement? The Roles of Persistence and Action Planning," *Motivation and Emotion* 43, no. 2 (2019): 205–17, https://doi.org/10.1007/s11031–018–9720–4.
4. "18 Ways to Cope with Frustration," Mental Health America, accessed January 29, 2023, https://mhanational.org/18-ways-cope-frustration.
5. Robin Sweetser, "What Weeds Tell You about Your Soil," *Old Farmer's Almanac*, updated December 3, 2022, https://www.almanac.com/what-weeds-tell-you-about-your-soil.
6. APA Dictionary of Psychology, s.v. "fear."
7. New Testament Greek Lexicon: King James Version, s.v. "elpis," Bible Study Tools, accessed April 26, 2023, https://www.biblestudytools.com/lexicons/greek/kjv/elpis.html.
8. "Fertilizer 101: The Big 3—Nitrogen, Phosphorus and Potassium," The Fertilizer Institute, May 7, 2014, https://www.tfi.org/the-feed/fertilizer-101-big-3-nitrogen-phosphorus-and-potassium.
9. *Strong's Concordance*, s.v. "apopnigó," Bible Hub, accessed April 28, 2023, https://biblehub.com/greek/638.htm.
10. Mark R. McMinn, *Why Sin Matters: The Surprising Relationship Between Our Sin and God's Grace* (Wheaton, IL: Tyndale House Publishers, 2004), 107.
11. Though researchers have identified multiple subcategories within the main soil types, four primary categories are widely accepted. See, for example, "Types of Soil," BYJU's Learning, accessed January 4, 2023, https://byjus.com/biology/types-of-soil/.

12. *Merriam–Webster Dictionary*, s.v. "loam," accessed December 21, 2022, https://www.merriam-webster.com/dictionary/loam.

13. Manjula V. Nathan, "Soils, Plant Nutrition and Nutrient Management," Extension, University of Missouri, accessed January 29, 2023, https://extension.missouri.edu/publications/mg4.

14. Luke Gatiboni, "Soils and Plant Nutrients," in *North Carolina Extension Gardener Handbook*, ed. K. A. Moore and L. K. Bradley (Raleigh: NC State Extension Publications, 2022), https://content.ces.ncsu.edu/extension-gardener-handbook/1-soils-and-plant-nutrients.

Chapter 5: How Does Your Garden Grow?

1. *Tab Time*, season 1, episode 1, "How Things Grow," produced by Tabitha Brown, published December 1, 2021, YouTube video, 22:34, https://youtu.be/zUTZEk32tc8.

2. Erika Krull, "Grief by the Numbers: Facts and Statistics," The Recovery Village Drug and Alcohol Rehab, May 26, 2022, https://www.therecoveryvillage.com/mental-health/grief/grief-statistics/.

3. "WHO COVID-19 Dashboard," World Health Organization, accessed April 19, 2023, https://covid19.who.int.

4. Damian F. Santomauro et al., "Global Prevalence and Burden of Depressive and Anxiety Disorders in 204 Countries and Territories in 2020 Due to the COVID-19 Pandemic," *The Lancet* 398, no. 10312 (November 2021): 1700–12, https://doi.org/10.1016/S0140–6736(21)02143–7.

5. Helen Huiskes, "It Takes a Campus: Pandemic Expands Mental Health Resources at Christian Colleges," *Christianity Today*, December 17, 2021, https://www.christianitytoday.com/news/2021/december/christian-college-mental-health-counseling-pandemic-demand.html.

6. "38% of U.S. Pastors Have Thought About Quitting Full-Time Ministry in the Past Year," Barna, November 16, 2021, https://www.barna.com/research/pastors-well-being/.

7. Peter Scazzero, *Emotionally Healthy Spirituality: It's Impossible to Be Spiritually Mature, While Remaining Emotionally Immature* (Grand Rapids, MI: Zondervan, 2017), 9, 44.

8. Scazzero, *Emotionally Healthy Spirituality*, 44.

9. Cynthia J. Price and Carole Hooven, "Interoceptive Awareness Skills for Emotion Regulation: Theory and Approach of Mindful Awareness in Body-Oriented Therapy (MABT)," *Frontiers in Psychology* 9 (May 2018): 798, https://doi.org/10.3389/fpsyg.2018.00798.

10. "How and Why to Practice Self-Care," Mental Health First Aid, March 14, 2022, https://www.mentalhealthfirstaid.org/2022/03/how-and-why-to-practice-self-care/.

Chapter 6: Water, Water Everywhere

1. Jack Gilbert, "Soil Health and Human Health: Microbial Diversity Helps Both," lecture, Nobel Conference: Living Soils: A Universe Underfoot, streamed live by Gustavus Adolphus College on October 3, 2018, YouTube video, 58:28, https://youtu.be/YWcFapREHnc.
2. APA Dictionary of Psychology, s.v. "belief."
3. APA Dictionary of Psychology, s.v. "thought."
4. Ziyan Yang et al., "Meaning Making Helps Cope with COVID-19: A Longitudinal Study," *Personality and Individual Differences* 174 (May 2021): 110670, https://www.ncbi.nlm.nih.gov/pmc/articles/PMC7825907/.
5. Judith E. Appel et al., "Meaning Violations, Religious/Spiritual Struggles, and Meaning in Life in the Face of Stressful Life," *International Journal for the Psychology of Religion* 30, no. 1 (May 2019): 1–17, PDF, https://spiritualitymeaningandhealth.uconn.edu/wp-content/uploads/sites/2598/2021/03/Meaning-Violations-ReligiousSpiritual-Struggles-and-Meaning-in-Life-in-the-Face-of-Stressful-Life-Events.pdf.
6. APA Dictionary of Psychology, s.v. "behavior."
7. APA Dictionary of Psychology, s.v. "private event."
8. New Testament Greek Lexicon: King James Version, s.v. "karpos," Bible Study Tools, accessed April 20, 2023, https://www.biblestudytools.com/lexicons/greek/kjv/karpos.html.
9. "Where Does a Plant's Mass Come From?," Arizona State University, accessed January 7, 2023, https://askabiologist.asu.edu/recipe-plant-growth.
10. Jun Zhan, Shuang Jiang, and Jing Luo, "The Angrier or the Happier the More Creative? The Impact of Anger and Joy Induction on Creative Problem-Solving and Divergent Thinking," *PsyCh Journal* 9, no. 6 (2020): 864–76, https://doi.org/10.1002/pchj.400.
11. Matthijs Baas, Carsten K. De Dreu, and Bernard A. Nijstad, "When Prevention Promotes Creativity: The Role of Mood, Regulatory Focus, and Regulatory Closure," *Journal of Personality and Social Psychology* 100, no. 5 (May 2011): 794–809, doi: 10.1037/a0022981.
12. Rajagopal Raghunathan and Michel Tuan Pham, "All Negative Moods Are Not Equal: Motivational Influences of Anxiety and Sadness on Decision Making," *Organizational Behavior and Human Decision Processes* 79, no. 1 (1999): 56–77, https://doi.org/10.1006/obhd.1999.2838.
13. Hou, Xuemin et al., "Water Transport in Fleshy Fruits: Research Advances, Methodologies, and Future Directions," *Physiologia Plantarum* 172, no. 4 (August 2021): 2203–16, https://doi.org/10.1111/ppl.13468.
14. Mlodinow, *Emotional*, xi.
15. Mlodinow, 19.

16. Mlodinow, 23.
17. Mlodinow, 73.

Chapter 7: Dust of the Ground

1. "What Is Dysautonomia?," National Institute of Neurological Disorders and Stroke, accessed April 20, 2023, https://www.ninds.nih.gov/health-information /disorders/dysautonomia.
2. "Nervous System—Touch," BBC Science, September 24, 2014, https://www.bbc .co.uk/science/humanbody/body/factfiles/touch/touch.shtml.
3. Leopold Eberhart et al., "Preoperative Anxiety in Adults—a Cross-Sectional Study on Specific Fears and Risk Factors," *BMC Psychiatry* 20, no. 1 (March 2020): 140, https://doi.org/10.1186/s12888–020–02552-w.
4. C. Nathan DeWall et al., "Acetaminophen Reduces Social Pain: Behavioral and Neural Evidence," *Psychological Science* 21, no. 7 (2010): 931–37, https://doi.org /10.1177/0956797610374741.
5. DeWall, "Acetaminophen Reduces Social Pain."
6. New Testament Greek Lexicon: King James Version, s.v. "ademoneo," Bible Study Tools, accessed April 20, 2023, https://www.biblestudytools.com/lexicons /greek/kjv/ademoneo.html.
7. New Testament Greek Lexicon: King James Version, s.v. "perilupos," Bible Study Tools, accessed April 20, 2023, https://www.biblestudytools.com/lexicons/greek /kjv/perilupos.html.
8. New Testament Greek Lexicon: King James Version, s.v. "ekthambeo," Bible Study Tools, accessed April 20, 2023, https://www.biblestudytools.com/lexicons /greek/kjv/ekthambeo.html.
9. New Testament Greek Lexicon: King James Version, s.v. "eulabeia," Bible Study Tools, accessed April 20, 2023, https://www.biblestudytools.com/lexicons/greek /kjv/eulabeia.html.
10. Raksha M. Patel and Stuti Mahajan, "Hematohidrosis: A Rare Clinical Entity," *Indian Dermatology Online Journal* 1, no. 1 (July–December 2010): 30–2, https:// doi.org/10.4103%2F2229–5178.73256.
11. 1 Kings 9:3; 2 Kings 20:5; 2 Chron. 7:12; Ps. 6:9; 66:19; Isa. 38:5; Luke 1:13; Acts 10:31.
12. New Testament Greek Lexicon: King James Version, s.v. "soma," Bible Study Tools, accessed June 22, 2023, https://www.biblestudytools.com/lexicons/greek/ nas/soma.html.
13. This definition was developed by Dr. Raja Selvam, a psychologist who specializes in embodying emotions. More information can be found in his book *The Practice of Embodying Emotions: A Guide for Improving Cognitive, Emotional, and Behavioral Outcomes* (Berkeley, CA: North Atlantic Books, 2022).

14. National Institute on Drug Abuse, ed. "Genetics and Epigenetics of Addiction Drug Facts," National Institutes of Health, June 2, 2023, https://nida.nih.gov/publications/drugfacts/genetics-epigenetics-addiction.
15. Antje Gentsch and Esther Kuehn, "Clinical Manifestations of Body Memories: The Impact of Past Bodily Experiences on Mental Health," *Brain Sciences* 12, no. 5 (May 2022): 594, https://www.ncbi.nlm.nih.gov/pmc/articles/PMC9138975/.
16. Rob Kurzban, "Why Can't You Hold Your Breath Until You're Dead?," *Evolutionary Psychology Blog*, February 7, 2011, archived at https://web.sas.upenn.edu/kurzbanepblog/2011/02/07/why-cant-you-hold-your-breath-until-youre-dead/.
17. Deb Dana, *Polyvagal Exercises for Safety and Connection: 50 Client-Centered Practices* (New York: W. W. Norton & Company, 2020), 2.
18. Sarah Sperber, "Fight or Flight Response: Definition, Symptoms, and Examples," Berkeley Well-Being Institute, accessed April 20, 2023, https://www.berkeleywellbeing.com/fight-or-flight.html.

Chapter 8: Shaky Ground

1. "Trauma and Violence," Substance Abuse and Mental Health Services Administration, updated September 27, 2022, https://www.samhsa.gov/trauma-violence.
2. "How to Manage Trauma," The National Council for Behavioral Health, August 2022, PDF, https://www.thenationalcouncil.org/wp-content/uploads/2022/08/Trauma-infographic.pdf.
3. C. Benjet et al., "The Epidemiology of Traumatic Event Exposure Worldwide: Results from the World Mental Health Survey Consortium," *Psychological Medicine* 46, no. 2 (2016): 327–43, https://doi.org/10.1017%2FS0033291715001981.
4. Angela Sweeney et al., "A Paradigm Shift: Relationships in Trauma-Informed Mental Health Services," BJPsych Advances 24, no. 5 (September 2018): 319–33, https://doi.org/10.1192/bja.2018.29.
5. SAMHSA, "Chapter 2: Trauma Awareness," in *Trauma-Informed Care in Behavioral Health Services*, Treatment Improvement Protocol 57 (Rockville, MD: Substance Abuse and Mental Health Services Administration, 2014), subheading "Mass Trauma," https://www.ncbi.nlm.nih.gov/books/NBK207203/.
6. SAMHSA, subheading "Mass Trauma."
7. SAMHSA, subheading "Trauma Affecting Communities and Cultures."
8. SAMHSA, subheading "Historical Trauma."
9. Robert W. Levenson, "The Autonomic Nervous System and Emotion," *Emotion Review* 6, no. 2 (2014): 100–12, https://doi.org/10.1177/1754073913512003.
10. Phillip Low, "Overview of the Autonomic Nervous System," *Merck Manual*, September 2022, https://www.merckmanuals.com/home/brain,-spinal-cord,-and

-nerve-disorders/autonomic-nervous-system-disorders/overview-of-the
-autonomic-nervous-system.

11. APA Dictionary of Psychology, s.v. "emotional regulation."

12. Kobe Campbell, *Why Am I Like This?: How to Break Cycles, Heal from Trauma, and Restore Your Faith* (Nashville: Thomas Nelson, 2023), 119.

13. Peter A. Levine, "Somatic Experiencing (SE)," Ergos Institute of Somatic Education, accessed December 26, 2022, https://www.somaticexperiencing.com /somatic-experiencing.

14. "What Is EMDR?," EMDR Institute, accessed May 23, 2023, https://www .emdr.com/what-is-emdr/.

Chapter 9: Wilderness

1. Bernice A. Pescosolido et al., "Trends in Public Stigma of Mental Illness in the US, 1996–2018," *JAMA Network Open* 4, no. 12 (2021): e2140202, https://doi .org/10.1001/jamanetworkopen.2021.40202.

2. "Mental Health," World Health Organization, June 17, 2022, https://www.who .int/news-room/fact-sheets/detail/mental-health-strengthening-our-response.

3. "What Is Mental Illness?," American Psychiatric Association, accessed April 20, 2023, https://www.psychiatry.org/patients-families/what-is-mental-illness.

4. Mark S. Salzer, Eugene Brusilovskiy, and Greg Townley, "National Estimates of Recovery-Remission From Serious Mental Illness," *Psychiatric Services* 69, no. 5 (2018): 523–28, https://doi.org/10.1176/appi.ps.201700401.

5. American Psychiatric Association, *Diagnostic and Statistical Manual of Mental Disorders*, 5th ed., text revision (Washington, DC: American Psychiatric Publishers, 2022).

6. "What Is Posttraumatic Stress Disorder (PTSD)?," American Psychiatric Association, accessed April 26, 2023, https://www.psychiatry.org/patients -families/ptsd/what-is-ptsd.

7. "What Is Posttraumatic Stress Disorder (PTSD)?," American Psychiatric Association.

8. NIMH, "What Is Post-Traumatic Stress Disorder, or PTSD?," National Institute of Mental Health, accessed June 21, 2023, https://www.nimh.nih.gov/health /publications/post-traumatic-stress-disorder-ptsd.

9. Levenson, "Autonomic Nervous System."

Chapter 10: The Wisdom of Trees

1. Tina Fossella, "Human Nature, Buddha Nature: On Spiritual Bypassing, Relationship, and the Dharma—an interview with John Welwood," John Welwood (website), accessed April 20, 2023, PDF, https://www.johnwelwood .com/articles/TRIC_interview_uncut.pdf.

2. Matt. 7:16–20.

Chapter 11: A Tree in the Temple

1. 1 Chron. 1:18.
2. Ali M. Alshami, "Pain: Is It All in the Brain or the Heart?," *Current Pain and Headache Reports* 23, no. 12 (November 2019): 88, https://pubmed.ncbi.nlm.nih .gov/31728781/.
3. Dana, *Polyvagal Exercises*, 7.
4. Dana, 10.
5. Low, "Overview of the Autonomic Nervous System."
6. Cynthia J. Price and Carole Hooven, "Interoceptive Awareness Skills for Emotion Regulation: Theory and Approach of Mindful Awareness in Body-Oriented Therapy (MABT)," *Frontiers in Psychology* 9, no. 798 (May 2018), https://doi.org/10.3389/fpsyg.2018.00798.
7. Victoria Weinblatt, "How Tree Roots Affect Soil," Week&, updated August 12, 2022, https://www.weekand.com/home-garden/article/tree-roots-affect-soil -18050740.php.
8. Jonathon Engels, "The Importance of Trees in the Garden," Permaculture News, March 3, 2017, https://www.permaculturenews.org/2017/03/03/importance-trees -garden/.

Chapter 12: Healing the Broken Heart

1. Adam Grant, "There's a Name for the Blah You're Feeling: It's Called Languishing," *New York Times*, April 19, 2021, https://www.nytimes.com/2021 /04/19/well/mind/covid-mental-health-languishing.html.
2. CDC, "Heart Disease and Mental Health Disorders," Centers for Disease Control and Prevention, accessed December 22, 2022, https://www.cdc.gov /heartdisease/mentalhealth.htm.
3. APA Dictionary of Psychology, s.v. "loneliness."
4. Dana, *Polyvagal Exercises*, 98.
5. Michelle Kroll, "Prolonged Social Isolation and Loneliness Are Equivalent to Smoking 15 Cigarettes a Day," University of New Hampshire (blog), May 2, 2022, https://extension.unh.edu/blog/2022/05/prolonged-social-isolation -loneliness-are-equivalent-smoking-15-cigarettes-day.
6. Dacher Keltner, "Hands On Research: The Science of Touch," *Greater Good*, September 29, 2010, https://greatergood.berkeley.edu/article/item/hands_on _research.
7. Keltner, "Hands On Research."
8. Susanna Newsonen, "The Shocking Truth About Hugs," *Psychology Today*, March 3, 2022, https://www.psychologytoday.com/us/blog/the-path-passionate -happiness/202203/the-shocking-truth-about-hugs.
9. APA Dictionary of Psychology, s.v. "grief."
10. Stephanie Hairston, "How Grief Shows Up in Your Body," WebMD, July 11,

2019, https://www.webmd.com/special-reports/grief-stages/20190711/how-grief
-affects-your-body-and-mind.

11. APA Dictionary of Psychology, s.v. "grief."

12. Associated Press, "A Brokenhearted Husband Dies After His Wife Is Killed in the Texas School Shooting," NPR, May 26, 2022, https://www.npr.org/2022/05 /26/1101682046/brokenhearted-husband-dies-wife-killed-texas-school-shooting.

13. "Takotsubo Cardiomyopathy," British Heart Foundation, last reviewed October 2019, https://www.bhf.org.uk/informationsupport/conditions /cardiomyopathy/takotsubo-cardiomyopathy.

14. APA Dictionary of Psychology, s.v. "anticipatory grief."

15. APA Dictionary of Psychology, s.v. "disenfranchised grief."

16. Nedra Glover Tawwab, "Love, Loss, & Learning to Grieve," Nedra Nuggets, March 1, 2023, https://nedratawwab.substack.com/p/love-loss-and-learning-to -grieve.

17. Susan Cain, *Bittersweet: How Sorrow and Longing Make Us Whole* (New York: Penguin Books, 2022), 10–11.

Chapter 13: Freeing the Angry Heart

1. "Serotonin," Cleveland Clinic, accessed April 26, 2023, https://my.clevelandclinic .org/health/articles/22572-serotonin.

2. Luca Passamonti et al., "Effects of Acute Tryptophan Depletion on Prefrontal-Amygdala Connectivity While Viewing Facial Signals of Aggression," *Biological Psychiatry* 71, no. 1 (2012): 36–43 https://doi.org/10.1016/j.biopsych.2011.07.033.

3. Michael O. Schroeder, "The Physical and Mental Toll of Being Angry All the Time," *U.S. News & World Report*, October 26, 2017, https://health.usnews.com /wellness/mind/articles/2017–10–26/the-physical-and-mental-toll-of-being -angry-all-the-time.

4. Schroeder, "Physical and Mental Toll."

5. Malek Mneimne, Amanda Kutz, and K. Lira Yoon, "Individual Differences in the Motivational Direction of Anger," *Personality and Individual Differences* 119 (December 2017): 56–59, https://www.sciencedirect.com/science/article/abs/pii /S0191886917304257.

Chapter 14: Calming the Fearful Heart

1. APA Dictionary of Psychology, s.v. "fear."

2. Harvard Medical School, "Understanding the Stress Response," Harvard Health Publishing, July 6, 2020, https://www.health.harvard.edu/staying-healthy /understanding-the-stress-response.

3. Dr. Russell Kennedy, *Anxiety RX: A New Prescription for Anxiety Relief from the Doctor Who Created It* (Sioux Falls, SD: Awaken Village Press, 2020), 167.

4. Jaime Rosenberg, "The Effects of Chronic Fear on a Person's Health," *American Journal of Managed Care* (blog), November 11, 2017, https://www.ajmc.com/view/the-effects-of-chronic-fear-on-a-persons-health.

5. Arko Banerjee et al., "Anxiety and Depression in Irritable Bowel Syndrome," *Indian Journal of Psychological Medicine* 39, no. 6 (November–December 2017): 741–45, https://doi.org/10.4103/ijpsym.ijpsym_46_17.

Chapter 15: Tending Your Embodied Garden

1. Gen. 3:16; Rom. 8:2.

2. Catherine A. Palmer, and Candice A. Alfano, "Sleep and Emotion Regulation: An Organizing, Integrative Review," *Sleep Medicine Reviews* 31 (2017): 6-16, https://doi.org/10.1016/j.smrv.2015.12.006.

3. Andrea Carretero-Krug, et al. "Hydration Status, Body Composition, and Anxiety Status in Aeronautical Military Personnel from Spain: A Cross-Sectional Study," *Military Medical Research* 8, no. 1 (2021): 35., https://doi.org/10.1186/s40779-021-00327-2.

4. Raza Ahmad, "How Much Water Do You Need Each Day?," *Health and Wellness* (blog), Penn Medicine, May 20, 2015, https://www.pennmedicine.org/updates/blogs/health-and-wellness/2015/may/how-much-water-do-you-need-each-day.

5. "Scheduled Eating: Why It's Beneficial and How to Start," Center for Healthy Eating and Activity, March 27, 2020, https://chear.ucsd.edu/blog/scheduled-eating-why-its-beneficial-and-how-to-start.

From War to Peace

1. Quoted in Patricia Harris, "Hearing the Voices of Those Who Are Educating for Shalom: What They Are Saying About Institutional Vision, Missional Goals, and Educational Models" (EdD diss., George Fox University, 2013), https://digitalcommons.georgefox.edu/cgi/viewcontent.cgi?article=1017&context=edd.

2. Harris, "Hearing the Voices."

3. Daniel L. Brunner, Jennifer L. Butler, and A. J. Swoboda, *Introducing Evangelical Ecotheology: Foundations in Scripture, Theology, History, and Praxis* (Grand Rapids, MI: Baker Publishing, 2014), 23.

4. James O'Donnell, "St. Augustine," *Encyclopedia Britannica*, last updated May 17, 2023, https://www.britannica.com/biography/Saint-Augustine.

5. Augustine, "Sermon 68" in *Sermons*, vol. 3, *Sermons 51–94*, trans. Edmund Hill, ed. John E. Rotelle (Hyde Park, NY: New City Press, 1991), 225.